A Parent's Guide to Healthy Children

From Preconception to Early Childhood

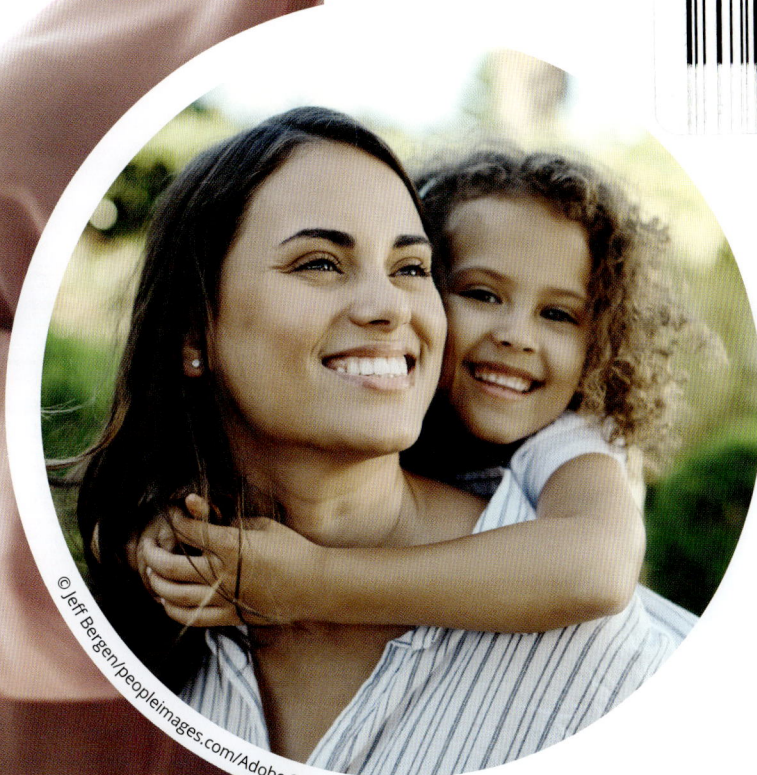

Children's
Health Defense

Visit our website at www.skyhorsepublishing.com.

10 9 8 7 6 5 4 3 2 1

Library of Congress Cataloging-in-Publication Data is available on file.

ISBN: 978-1-64821-193-5
eBook ISBN: 978-1-64821-196-6

Cover design by Children's Health Defense
Photos from Adobe Stock

Printed in the United States of America

Table of Contents

Introduction 1

Chapter One: Preconception Planning 3

  The Seed 4

  Factors Affecting Fertility 5

  Optimal Nutrition for Preconception, Pregnancy, and Postpartum 6

  Foods to Avoid During Preconception 12

  Minimizing Exposure to Environmental Toxins 13

Chapter Two: What Happens During Pregnancy? 15

  Mind, Body, and Spirit 16

  Common Discomforts During Pregnancy 18

  Vaccination During Pregnancy 24

Chapter Three: Planning for Childbirth 29

  Exploring Childbirth Options 30

  The Rise of Hospital Births 31

  Hospital Birth Today 32

  Home Birth 35

  Birth Centers 36

  Natural Interventions During Labor and Delivery 37

  Support During Childbirth 38

  Day-of-Birth Medical Interventions 39

Chapter Four: The First Year 43

  Therapeutic Touch 44

  The Infant Gut Microbiome and the Benefits of Breastfeeding 45

  Antibiotics and the Microbiome 47

  Breastfeeding Challenges and Alternatives 49

  Gastroesophageal Reflux 53

  Newborn Reflexes 55

  Infant Breathing 57

  Sleeping: When and Where 60

  Vaccination Risks 62

  Skin: The Largest Organ 65

  Maternal Changes 67

  Postpartum Depression 68

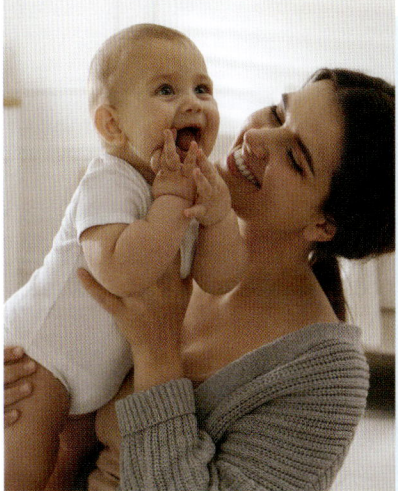

© New Africa/Adobe Stock

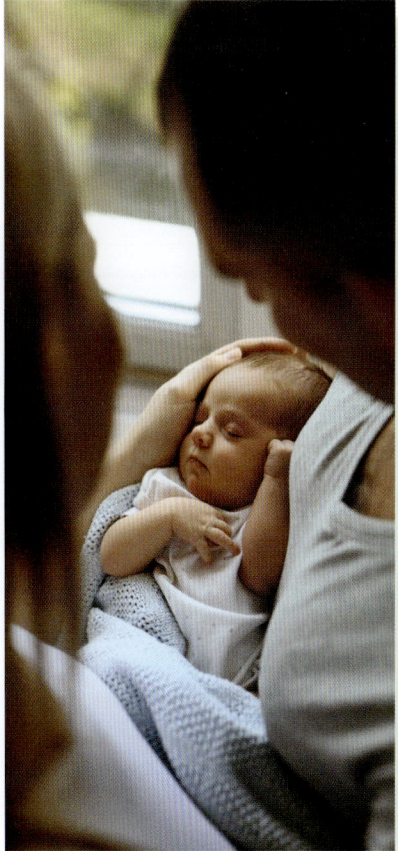

© Inna Ylasova/Adobe Stock

Chapter Five: The Solid Food Transition 71

Introducing Solid Food....................................71

Food Reactions and Food Allergies 75

Chapter Six: Developmental Milestones 78

Teaching and Learning: The Joy of Communication 80

Anticipating and Responding to a Child's Needs..........81

Children Set the Pace....................................83

Developmental Milestones 85

Developmental Delays and the 2022
Revised Developmental Milestones 89

Vaccine Ingredients as Environmental Toxins.............97

Chapter Seven: Environmental Exposures...............99

Synthetic Chemicals 100

Neurotoxic Metals 102

Fluoride 106

Electromagnetic Fields (EMFs) 108

Chapter Eight: Childhood Illness 109

Detoxification and Restoration 110

Medications and Warning Signs 112

Chapter Nine: Toys 113

The Importance of Imaginative Play 114

The First Few Years 114

Toys to Avoid 115

Better Options 115

Chapter Ten: Safety Tips.............................116

Babyproofing the Home 116

Car Seats and Strollers................................118

Choking and Accidental Ingestion.......................119

Other Potential Child Hazards 119

Chapter Eleven: The Parenting Journey 120

Sleep 121

Exercise...122

Postpartum Nutrition 122

Social Support...123

A Journey..123

Appendix: Typical Developmental Milestones,
2 Months Through 4 Years of Age........................124

Endnotes 133

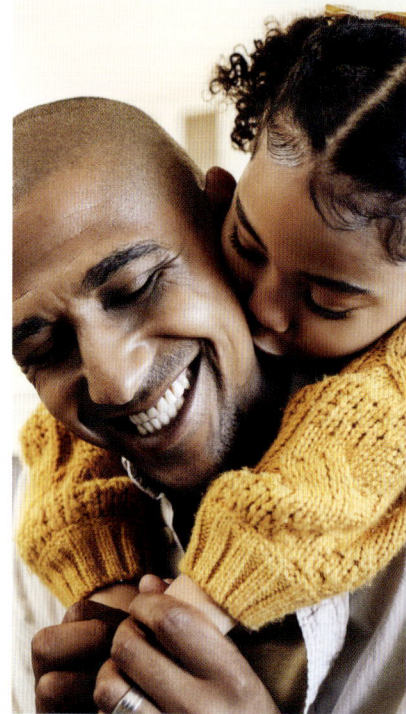

© Azee/peopleimages.com/Adobe Stock

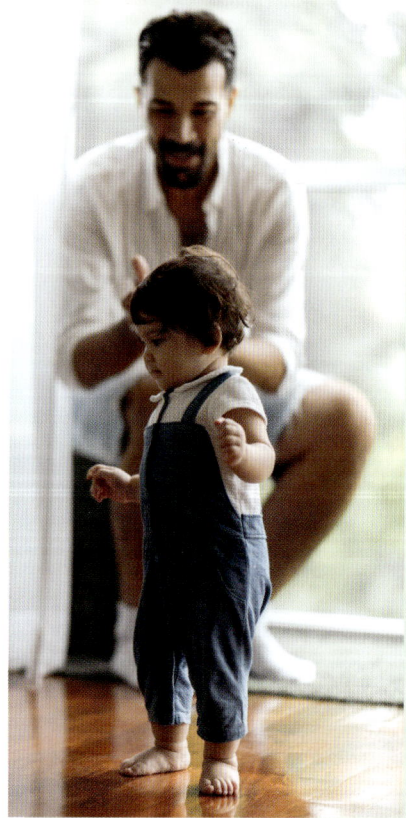

© Chokniti/Adobe Stock

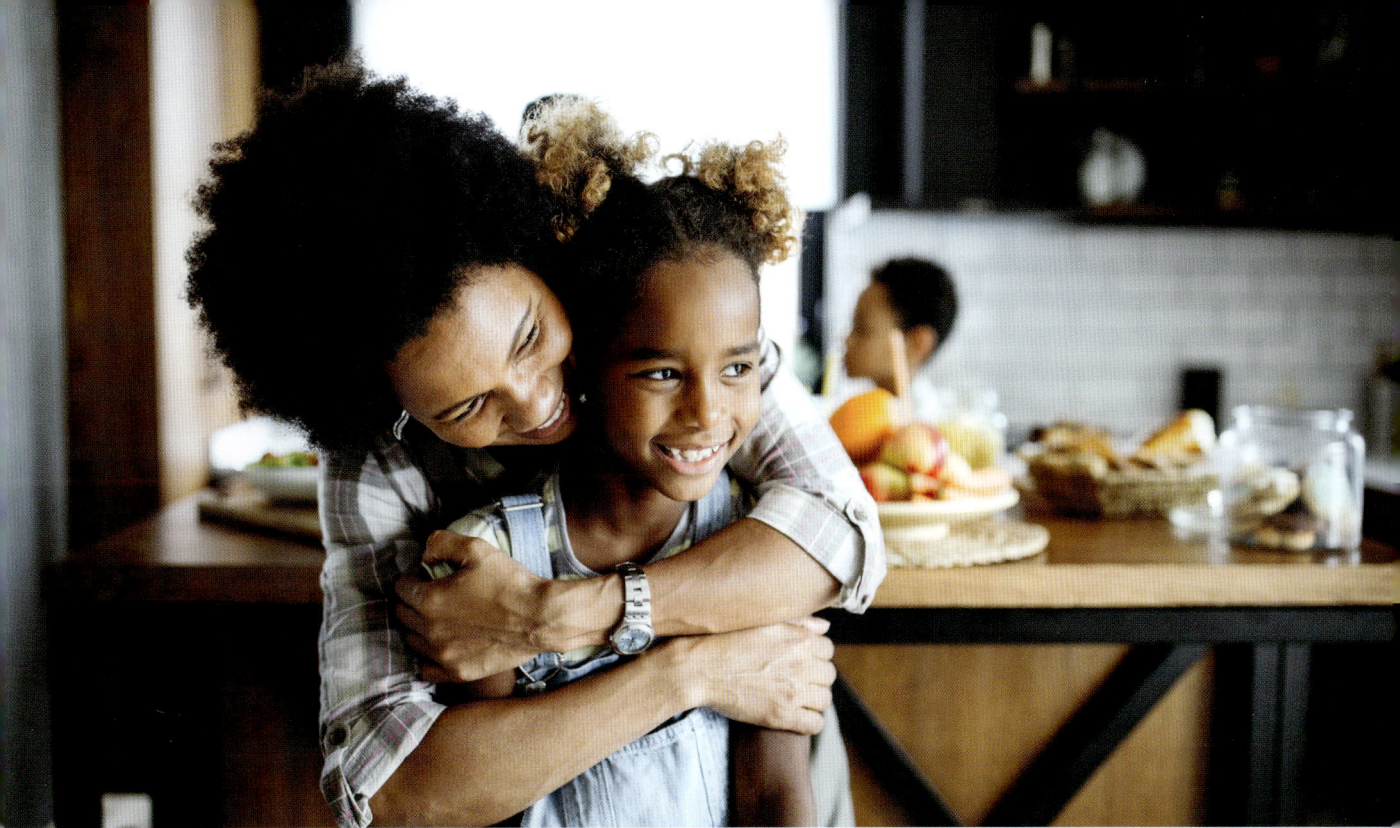

Introduction

This book is in defense of the child, and in defense of the freedom of parents and guardians to make health and wellness decisions for their children. Empowered and loving adults provide the foundation for children's healthy habits.[1] Parents have the innate ability to respond to their children in ways that promote health and vitality.

This time in history is unveiling some of the deepest inconsistencies in conventional Western medicine, both in the United States and around the world. It was only in the 19th and 20th centuries that practitioners of Western medicine began limiting their practice to knowledge of the physical body, gained through observation and experimentation. Before then, healing took into account the spiritual dimensions of health as well. Today, a growing number of people—both parents and professionals—recognize medicine's narrow focus on the physical as being detrimental to health and healing,[2] and they understand the importance of allowing children to grow up physically, mentally, emotionally, and spiritually healthy. The time is ripe for shifting the medical paradigm.

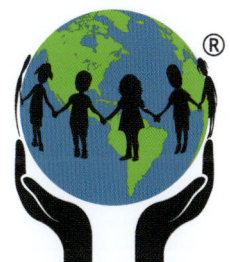

Over the last few years, people from all walks of life have experienced governmental and pharmaceutical overreach, negatively affecting their ability to make informed decisions regarding medical treatments, their right to bodily autonomy, and their right to full transparency. This has given rise to a powerful new movement of parents and caregivers committed to making health decisions and choices for themselves and their children without interference. Many parents also want to guide children so that young people:

- Trust their own ability to maintain and restore balance and health
- Understand simple steps they can take to maintain health and prevent and treat illness
- Grow up taking charge of their health and health care

Parents are their children's best advocates, and they must be able to make health decisions with confidence. No parent should ever feel vulnerable or victimized when they seek medical assistance for their child.[3] This eBook provides readers with resources they can use to support their children's health and the sometimes complex medical decisions that are unique to each child and family. Though shaped by medical, psychological, social, and cultural forces, parental decision-making should not be subject to pressure from outside influences. Instead, parents should be able to obtain support from trusted medical professionals who emphasize informed consent and risk-based analysis.

There is no need for parents to fear speaking up or to feel alone. All parents share a purpose: to protect the most precious generation and raise vibrant, healthy, and happy children.

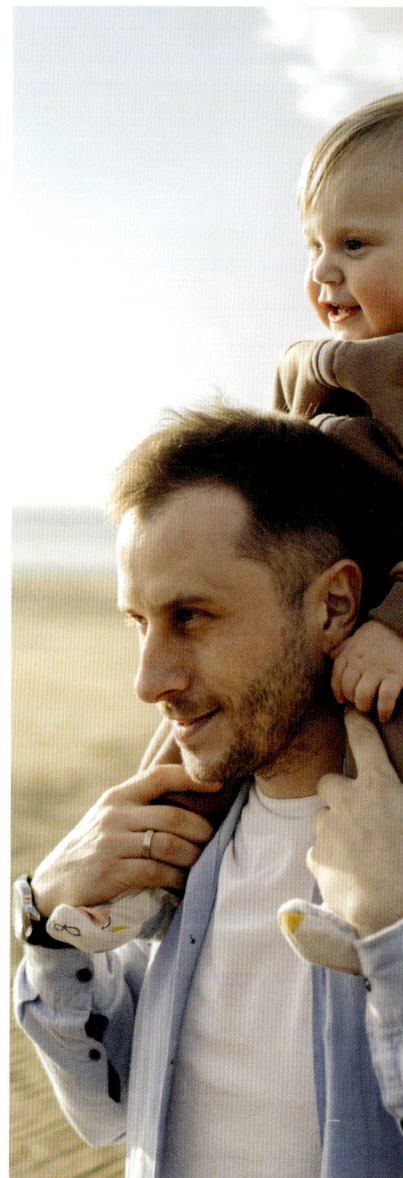

© muse studio/Adobe Stock

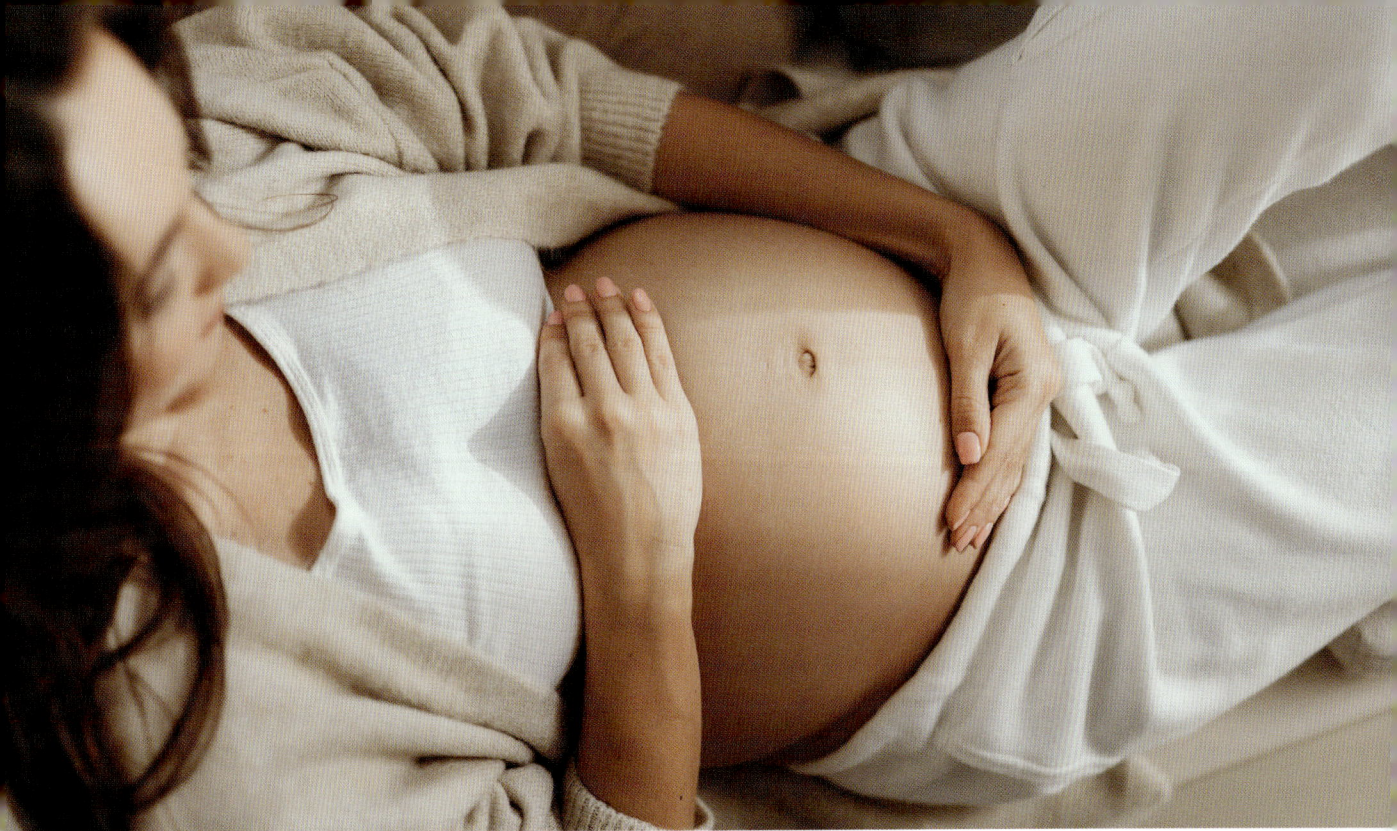

Chapter One: Preconception Planning

"If we hope to create a nonviolent world where respect and kindness replace fear and hatred, we must begin with how we treat others at the beginning of life. For that is where our deepest patterns are set. From these roots grow fear and alienation—or love and trust." — **Suzanne Arms**

For many years, author Suzanne Arms has challenged the status quo in terms of how society cares for childbearing women and brings babies into the world. According to Arms, society often fails to meet the needs of the mother-baby dyad and neglects children's proper brain and immune development.[4]

This inattention often starts even earlier, during preconception—the period before a woman gets pregnant.

However, as societal knowledge and ideas shift, even conventional medicine is evolving toward a focus that goes beyond merely "planting a seed" to emphasizing preconception planning. This perspective recognizes that baseline health and happiness at conception matter. Healthy women and men are the foundation on which society can cultivate healthy future generations.

> *Healthy women and men are the foundation on which society can cultivate healthy future generations.*

In this chapter, we will:

- Discuss factors that influence natural fertility
- Address daily stressors that may interfere with fertility
- Discuss the importance of reducing or eliminating preconception exposure to environmental toxins
- Explore health and nutrition options
- Share resources to facilitate support for future mothers embarking on this journey

The Seed

"I feel so alone; my partner and I are suffering from infertility. I have tried it all—I am in desperate need of quality support and guidance."

Unfortunately, subfertility and infertility are increasingly common. A variety of internal and external factors are contributing to this growing concern, with diagnoses of "unexplained infertility" on the rise. In the United States, an estimated one in five women aged 15 to 49 with no prior births fails to get pregnant after one year of trying; one in four reproductive-age women has difficulty either getting pregnant or carrying a pregnancy to term.[5] Both women and men can contribute to infertility, and it is important to consider the couple "as a unit."[6]

Conventional approaches to treating infertility—medication, injections, intrauterine insemination (IUI), or in vitro fertilization (IVF)—can be extremely stressful. Not only are these treatments expensive and rarely covered by health insurance, but they may not be for everyone.

Instead of or in addition to medications or IVF treatments, a holistic and integrative approach to fertility is an alternative worth considering. This approach encompasses the whole person, recognizing mind, body, spirit, emotions, and lifestyle as key factors that can maximize fertility—for both women and men. Specific interventions may include meditation, Chinese medicine, yoga, hypnosis, mitigation of stressors, dietary change, or supplementation. Chinese medicine practitioner Dr. Randine Lewis, whose book *The Infertility Cure* has helped numerous couples overcome fertility challenges,[7] emphasizes the importance of women getting to know their cycle and learning how to positively affect it. The goal is to focus more deeply on the overall health of the couple to increase the chances of conceiving naturally. As one author puts it, "the best way to be fertile and have a healthy baby is to have vibrant health."[8]

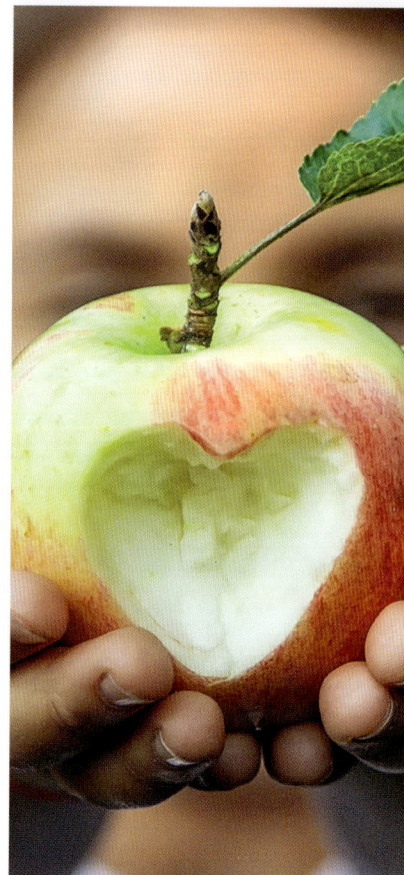

© yanadjan/Adobe Stock

> **One in four reproductive-age women has difficulty either getting pregnant or carrying a pregnancy to term.**

If infertility is a concern, we recommend consulting with a trusted provider who is willing to partner with future parents in the decision-making process and provide meaningful support and guidance. Fortunately, a growing number of holistic providers specialize in infertility treatment. Alternatives for Healing is a leading alternative medicine site for finding holistic and integrative medicine practitioners.[9] There are also virtual and in-person support groups that connect individuals facing infertility, such as the National Infertility Association's RESOLVE.[10] The fellowship of a support group allows individuals who share the same challenges to connect with one another and facilitates courage, strength, and hope.

Factors Affecting Fertility

"When a plant does not grow, you fix the environment that it's subjected to, not the plant."
— **Yashmayi Bhoi**

Couples wanting to conceive need to understand the basics about the female and male reproductive systems and the importance of timing, with the five days before and the day of ovulation being the "fertile window."[11] It also helps to trust that the mother's body—the home for the growing fetus—is designed to properly nourish and nurture a baby as long as it is treated gently and kindly, beginning during preconception. Paying attention to both female and male preconception health can help ensure that after conception, the baby will grow and flourish.

> *Paying attention to both female and male preconception health can help ensure that after conception, the baby will grow and flourish.*

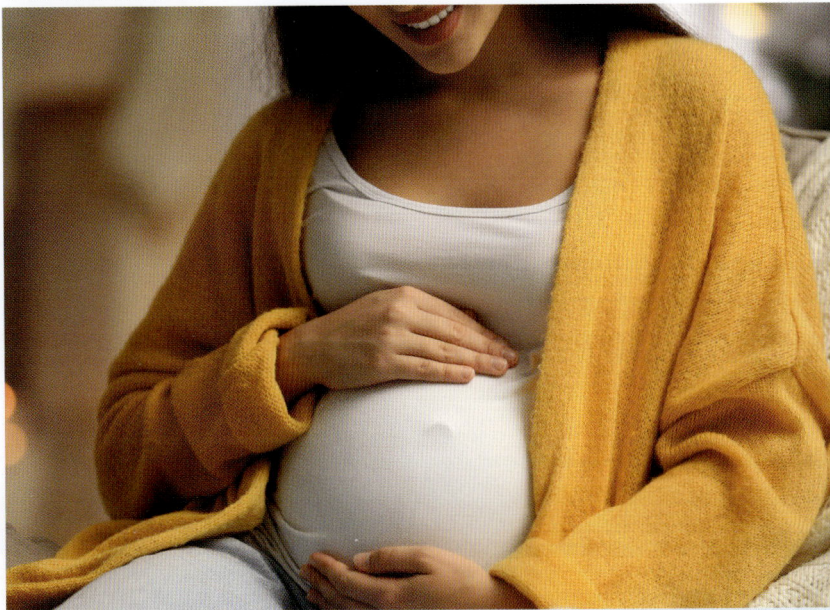

For women, conception requires a proper internal environment. Each woman has an innate body clock that relates directly to the reproductive system. Research shows that some causes of infertility may be directly related to disorders in this biological clock. For example, stress can cause an imbalance, while daily physical activity, wholesome nutrition, and other supports can aid in restoring balance. Low progesterone, high testosterone, low thyroid hormone, and insulin resistance are examples of imbalances that can affect ovulation and make it more difficult to get pregnant.[12] Women who have been on hormonal birth control for any length of time also may have more trouble conceiving; birth control pills also deplete nutrients "critical to the development of a healthy nervous system in future developing babies."[13]

The external environment is also important. For example, studies in mice show that cell phone radiation affects female "reproductive performance" through multiple mechanisms,[14] with multiple studies indicating that it "poses a serious hazardous health risk for women of childbearing age," affecting their ability "to conceive, carry and deliver healthy children."[15]

For men, exposure to environmental toxins, again including radiation from cell phones and laptops, can contribute to abnormal sperm or interfere with hormonal balance.[16] Other factors affecting male fertility include compromised baseline health status, older paternal age, poor nutrition, and stress.

Optimal Nutrition for Preconception, Pregnancy, and Postpartum

"Our food should be our medicine and our medicine should be our food." — **Hippocrates**

Recognizing that an egg takes three months to mature, preconception planning should begin six months in advance at a minimum,[17] with two years being even more ideal. Currently, nearly half of all pregnancies are unplanned, however, which can place the mother and infant at a greater risk for prenatal and postnatal complications. Whether a pregnancy is planned or unexpected, it is never too early or too late to make conscious dietary changes that provide for parents' and baby's optimal health.

> *Recognizing that an egg takes three months to mature, preconception planning should begin six months in advance at a minimum.*

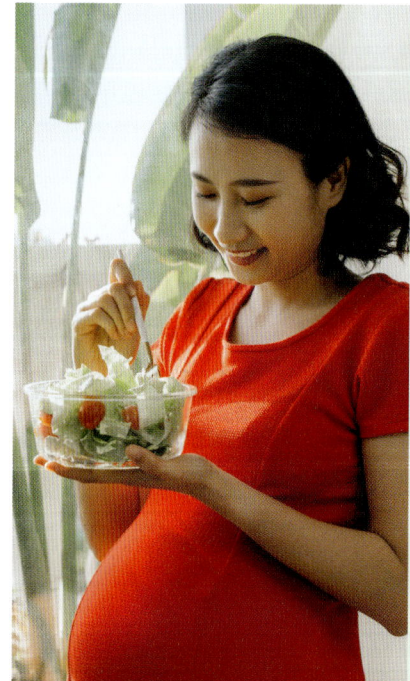

© makistock/Adobe Stock

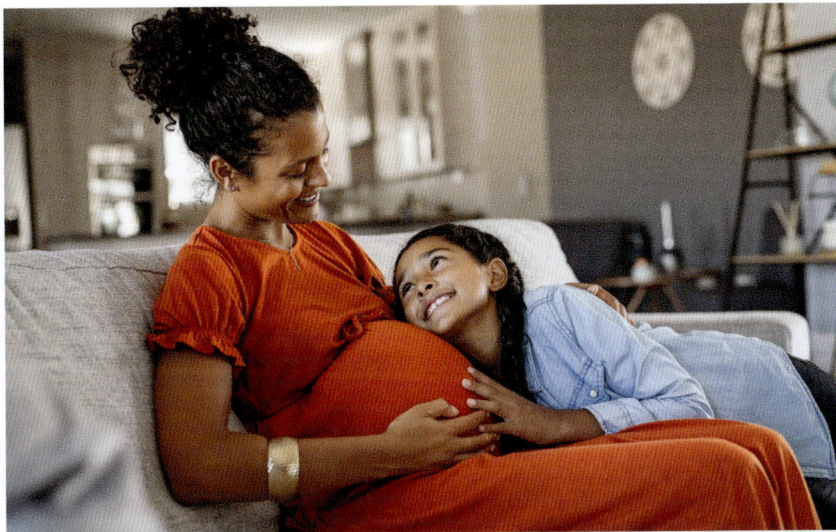

© Rido/Adobe Stock

A successful diet that supports fertility, pregnancy, and the needs of breastfeeding infants should emphasize whole fresh foods that are nutrient-dense.

Eating habits greatly influence both fertility and the health of a growing baby.[18] A successful diet that supports fertility, pregnancy, and the needs of breastfeeding infants should emphasize whole fresh foods that are nutrient-dense—including foods high in vitamins A, D, and K and minerals.[19] As Sally Fallon Morell, founder and president of the Weston A. Price Foundation (an organization "dedicated to restoring nutrient-dense foods to the human diet") puts it, "you need to have extra nutrition during that period of conception and growth because that never comes back. You only have one chance to get it right."[20]

To support fertility and a healthy pregnancy, couples should choose and consume high-quality foods that may include:

- A variety of organic, grass-fed meats
- Wild-caught seafood (such as cod, salmon, crab, shrimp, and fish eggs)
- Organic organ meats (such as chicken liver)
- Bone broths
- Organic pastured eggs and especially egg yolks
- Organic, grass-fed, and preferably raw dairy[21]
- Whole grains, soaked or sprouted to ensure proper digestion[22]
- Properly prepared (i.e., soaked or sprouted) nuts, seeds, and legumes
- A rainbow of organic, antioxidant-rich fruits and vegetables
- Sauerkraut, kimchi, and other fermented foods
- Organic berries
- Avocados
- Plentiful butter, ghee, other animal fats such as lard and tallow, coconut oil, and cold-pressed virgin olive oil

Animal foods rich in natural vitamin A—such as eggs, butter, cheese, liver, fish, and high-vitamin cod liver oil—are particularly important during preconception. Vitamin A is the "concertmaster of fetal development" and is essential for sending the signals that ensure formation of a healthy heart—a process that begins around three weeks of pregnancy, well before most women even know they are pregnant.[23] Vitamin A in the form of beta-carotene (called "provitamin A carotenoids") is present in orange vegetables such as carrots and sweet potatoes but absorbs poorly compared to the vitamin A in animal foods.[24]

Pregnant women sometimes encounter the message that too much vitamin A can be toxic, but it is important to understand that warnings about vitamin A toxicity are all based on synthetic forms of vitamin A in supplements. In fact, while synthetic retinyl palmitate is a known teratogen (something that causes fetal abnormalities),[25] "[n]atural food sources of vitamin A are well tolerated at even high doses."[26]

Also within a few weeks of conception—and again, before many women realize they are pregnant—the neural plate begins to fold inward, forming the neural tube that will eventually become the baby's brain and spinal cord. Defects in the fetal neural tube may cause abnormalities in the infant's brain and spine. Women can decrease the risk of neural tube defects with an adequate intake of folate and other essential vitamins and minerals. Foods rich in folate—liver, egg yolks, seafood, legumes, and leafy greens—as well as omega-3 fatty acids, iron, B-vitamins, choline, and vitamin A during preconception and pregnancy will provide the baby with the nutrients required for musculoskeletal and brain development (see the "Preconception, Pregnancy, and Postpartum" box on page 10).[27]

> *Defects in the fetal neural tube may cause abnormalities in the infant's brain and spine. Women can decrease the risk of neural tube defects with an adequate intake of folate and other essential vitamins and minerals.*

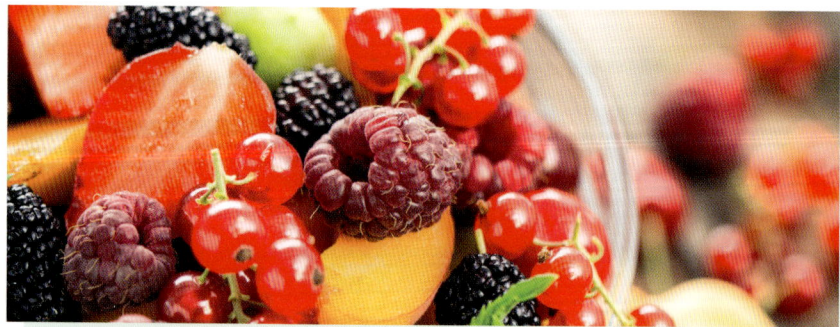

© pilipphoto/Adobe Stock

The Weston A. Price Foundation does not recommend prenatal vitamins, generally full of synthetic ingredients which are poorly absorbed and "don't come with the right kind of co-factors."[28] Prenatal vitamins are no substitute for a nutrient-dense diet. They also may contain synthetic food dyes or food colorings, synthetic retinyl palmitate, synthetic folic acid, monosodium glutamate (MSG), polyethylene glycol (PEG), bisphenol A (BPA), and/or GMO ingredients. The Foundation's "Diet for Pregnant and Nursing Mothers" provides guidelines for an optimal diet.[29]

The body has a particularly difficult time metabolizing the synthetic folic acid included in many prenatal supplements; moreover, synthetic folic acid does not cross the placenta.[30] Women who nevertheless choose to take a prenatal supplement should avoid those containing synthetic folic acid and look for a methylated folate like L-methylfolate (600 to 800 mcg of active folate daily).

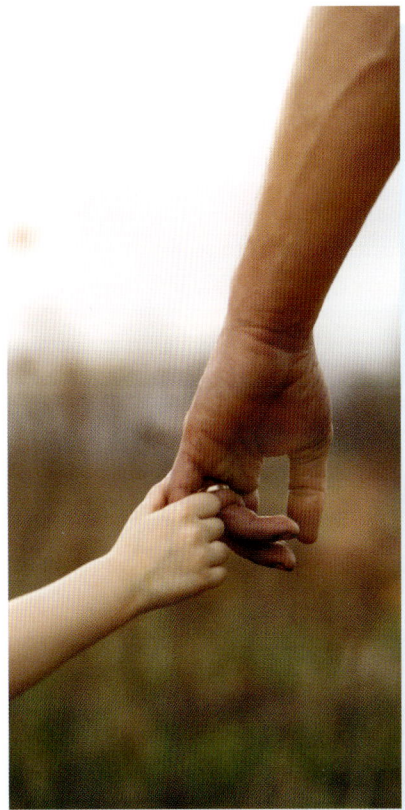

© Olga Simonova/Adobe Stock

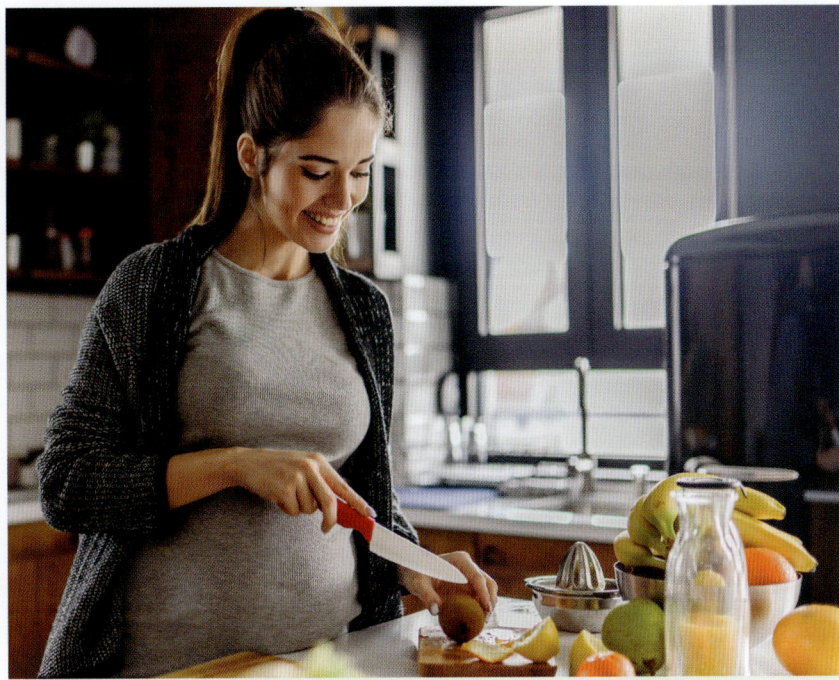

© lordn/Adobe Stock

" Prenatal vitamins are no substitute for a nutrient-dense diet. "

Preconception, Pregnancy, and Postpartum: Essential Vitamins and Minerals

- **Folate:** Folate, recommended three to six months prior to conception and during pregnancy, aids in protecting the rapidly dividing cells of the baby and is known for its important role in decreasing the risk of neural tube defects (brain and spinal defects) in infants. Food sources of folate include liver, legumes, egg yolks, seafood, and leafy greens.

- **Choline:** Choline (found in liver, egg yolks, grass-fed dairy, fish, meats, nuts, and some cruciferous vegetables) also provides support essential for spinal cord formation.

- **Vitamins A, D, and K:** Vitamins A, D (in the form of D3), and K work together synergistically. During the first few weeks of pregnancy, vitamin A from animal foods plays a vital role in healthy organ development; it is also important for immune system function, skin health, and eye development. Vitamin D3 facilitates sufficient calcium and phosphorus absorption; however, there is a limit to how much of this active form of vitamin D someone can absorb at once. Vitamin K plays an important role in bone formation. For all three, good sources include butter, egg yolks, and liver; other sources of vitamin K include hard and soft cheeses and a fermented form of soy called natto.

- **Vitamin B6 (pyridoxine):** Vitamin B6 supports the luteal phase that primes the maternal body for embryo implantation, and is essential for central nervous system development in the fetus. Women who have used oral contraceptives are at risk of a B6 deficiency. Animal food sources (e.g., liver, red meat, salmon and other fish, raw grass-fed milk and cheese) provide much higher bioavailability but are sensitive to overcooking.

> *During the first few weeks of pregnancy, vitamin A from animal foods plays a vital role in healthy organ development.*

© ltummy/Adobe Stock

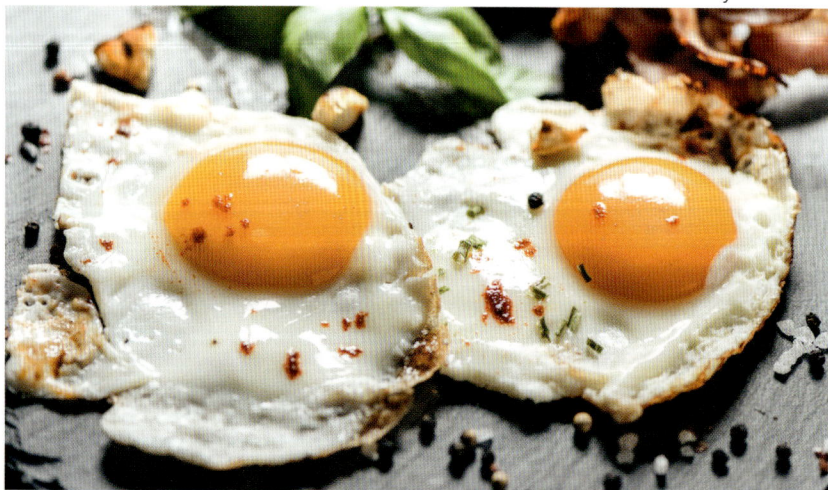

- **Vitamin B12 and Selenium:** Both boost fertility and mitigate the potential risk of miscarriage. Vitamin B12 is almost exclusively in animal foods (meat, organ meats, fish, shellfish, milk products). Supplementation with isolated B12 (but not B12 analogs, which can be harmful) may be indicated in individuals with severe deficiencies. As for selenium, sources include fish, shellfish, poultry, organ meats, Brazil nuts, and dairy products.

- **Vitamin C:** Vitamin C supports the immune system and helps the body make progesterone, needed for maintaining a healthy pregnancy. Heat-sensitive vitamin C is found in many fruits and vegetables and some animal organs.

- **Vitamin E:** Vitamin E protects maternal eggs from damage that could be caused by unstable molecules in the body and works in concert with trace minerals such as selenium and zinc. Sources include butter, organ meats, grains, nuts, seeds, legumes, and leafy green vegetables.

- **Calcium:** Calcium supports healthy bone growth; to be fully absorbed, the body also needs vitamin D3.

- **Copper and Zinc:** Copper aids in antioxidant production, but is only needed in minute amounts and is more effective when balanced with zinc. Zinc supports the body by making superoxide dismutase, an enzyme that helps keep maternal eggs healthy. Because the most reliable sources of zinc are eggs and red meat, individuals who eat plant-based diets are more likely to end up with copper-zinc imbalances.

- **Iodine:** Iodine plays a necessary role in making thyroid hormones; the thyroid is a vital hormone gland involved in metabolism, growth, and development.

- **Iron:** Iron supports a baby's development and is essential to build healthy blood cells, which deliver oxygen to mother and baby.

- **Magnesium:** Magnesium provides necessary support both for fertility and the health of the baby.

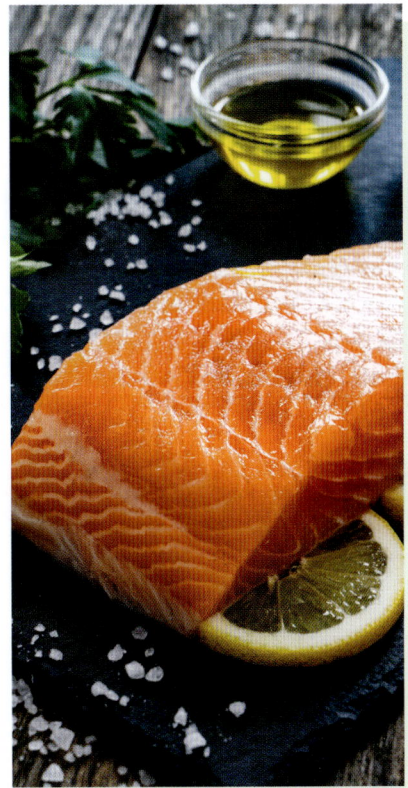

© Jacek Chabraszewski/Adobe Stock

> *Vitamin C supports the immune system and helps the body make progesterone, needed for maintaining a healthy pregnancy.*

Foods to Avoid During Preconception

During preconception, there are also foods that parents-to-be should avoid—such as fast foods and processed foods devoid of nutrition and laden with additives.[31] One study found that women who ate fast food at least four times a week had double the risk of infertility compared to women who never ate fast food.[32] The goal is to ensure that women and their partners are functioning at their highest potential to allow for conception.

Unsaturated trans fats may increase the risk of ovulatory infertility. In a study conducted in 2007, the risk of ovulatory infertility increased by more than 70% with every 2% increase in trans fat intake.[33]

Women trying to conceive should completely avoid certain types of fish at the top of the marine food chain, such as white (albacore) tuna, bigeye tuna, swordfish, marlin, orange roughy, king mackerel, shark, and tilefish from the Gulf of Mexico. These have the highest mercury levels. However, there is some evidence that eating fish with a higher concentration of selenium than mercury can help minimize mercury risks.[34]

Studies have linked diets high in sugar and refined carbohydrates with fertility difficulties.[35] Nutritionists recommend avoiding or substantially decreasing intake of sweetened sodas and juices. There is also evidence that artificial sweeteners—such as aspartame, acesulfame potassium (known as Ace-K), Splenda, sorbitol, Sweet'N Low®, and sucralose—pose health risks.[36] It would be wise to avoid beverages featuring these sweeteners.

There are also many reasons to avoid soy both during preconception and through the postpartum period, with evidence that "maternal consumption of soy products transfers estrogenic hormone disruptors to [the] fetus" and also to a breastfeeding infant: "Several hundred studies overwhelmingly conclude soy phyto-toxic causation of an assortment of severe, painful and often irreversible neurological and physiological disorders ... more often caused during developmental exposures."[37]

> *One study found that women who ate fast food at least four times a week had double the risk of infertility compared to women who never ate fast food.*

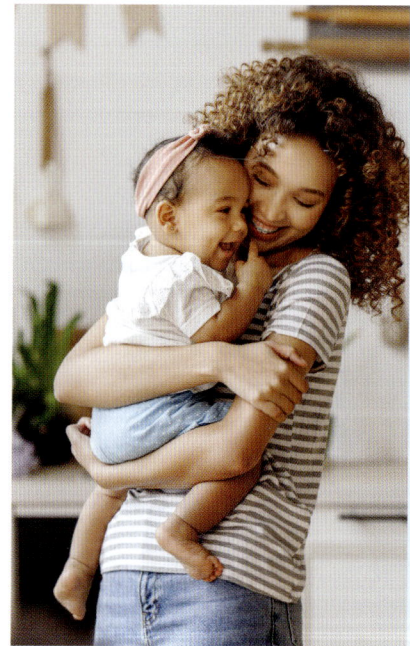

© JenkoAtaman/Adobe Stock

Research has established that consuming alcohol during pregnancy can cause a host of complications for the fetus, but the effects of alcohol on fertility are not as well studied.[38] An occasional drink will probably not have an impact on fertility. However, studies have linked excessive preconception alcohol intake to infertility in both women and men due to its potential to affect hormones adversely.[39,40]

After conception, maternal nutrition continues to play a vital role, ensuring that a baby will thrive prenatally and after birth. The foods that a mother consumes will strongly affect infant birth weight, gestational age, immune system functioning, and brain development. Neurodevelopmental processes occur rapidly during the estimated 280 days that a baby is growing in the womb.

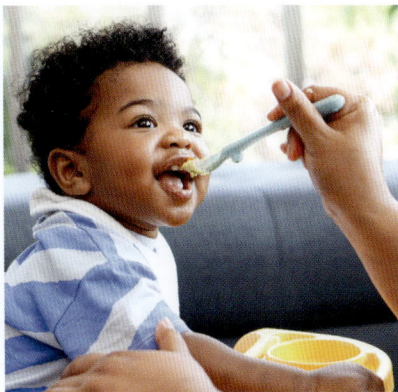

© SUPERMAO/Adobe Stock

Minimizing Exposure to Environmental Toxins

Exposures to environmental toxins can have a negative impact on fertility (see "Toxins and Fertility," p. 14), decreasing the odds of natural conception as well as lowering the success rate of infertility treatments.[41] As already noted, human fertility is declining worldwide. According to an article published in 2018 in *Integrative Medicine*, "While much of the 50% decrease in the number of children born per woman in the past 60 years is due to choice, an increasing number of couples—now 1 in 7 to 10 in North America—are have [sic] serious difficulty conceiving."[42] The study singled out the growing body burden of environmental toxins in both men and women as a "significant cause of this progressive loss of fertility." As described in the article, environmental toxins can cause infertility in four ways: endocrine disruption, damage to the female reproductive system, damage to the male reproductive system, and impaired fetal viability.

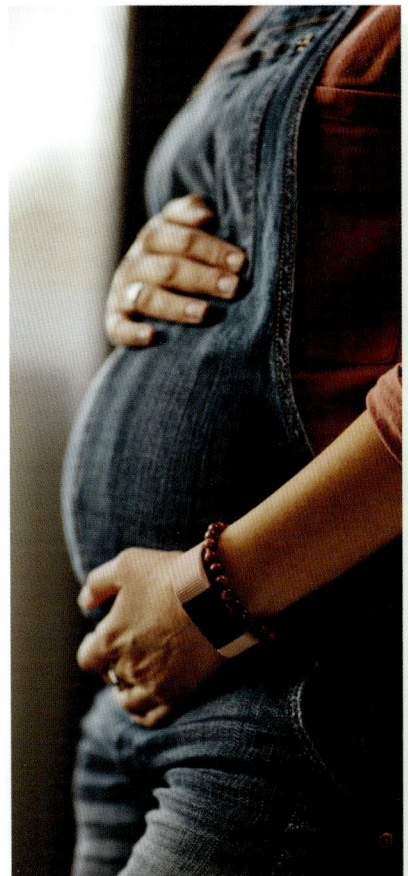

© Chika_milan/Adobe Stock

> *Neurodevelopmental processes occur rapidly during the estimated 280 days that a baby is growing in the womb.*

Toxins and Fertility

A wide range of environmental toxins encountered in personal care products, household cleaning products, textiles, food packaging, and non-stick products can disrupt fertility. These include:

- **Bisphenol A** (BPA) found in some food and drink packaging and hard plastic packaging

- **Phthalates** in soft plastic products

- **Parabens** and **benzophenones** in sunscreens and personal care products

- **Fire retardants** in electronics and furniture

- **Mercury** and **PCBs** (polychlorinated biphenyls) in fish such as tuna

- **Organochlorine compounds** such as chlorinated pesticides, PCBs, and dioxins present in many paper products

- **Organophosphate** pesticides and herbicides

- Other **pesticides** in conventionally farmed produce

- Additional chemicals, metals, and air pollutants

For more details on these environmental toxins, see Chapter Seven.

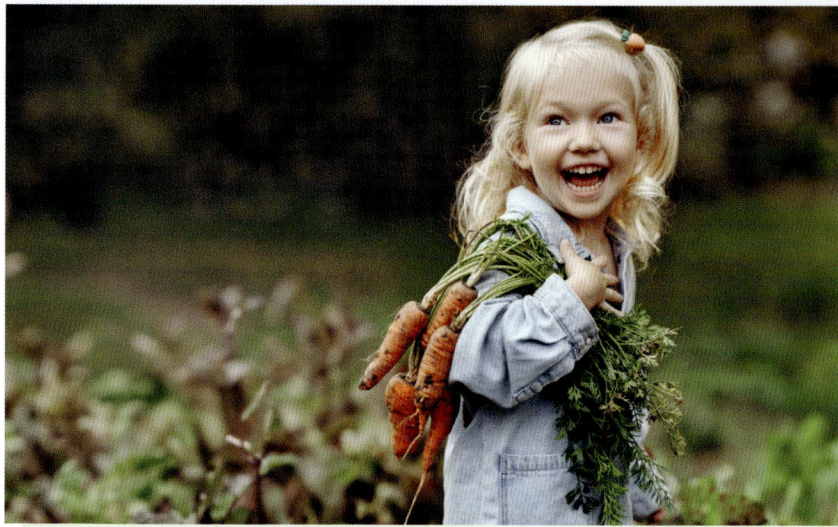

© Natalia Shmatova/Adobe Stock

Although it can be difficult to completely eliminate all toxic exposures, greater awareness can help in the selection of less toxic cleaning, laundry, and personal care options. However, this requires ascertaining the difference between products that are truly organic, nontoxic, and better for the environment and those that simply claim to be "natural" or "green." A staff scientist at the Natural Resources Defense Council (NRDC) states that terms like "natural," "green," and "nontoxic" are "unfortunately not regulated and are not legal definitions, so they don't really mean anything."[43] For cleaning products, the most effective solution can be to make them at home. This can be as simple as using white vinegar and baking soda, with the option of adding a little lemon, ginger, or orange essential oil.

> *A wide range of environmental toxins encountered in personal care products, household cleaning products, textiles, food packaging, and non-stick products can disrupt fertility.*

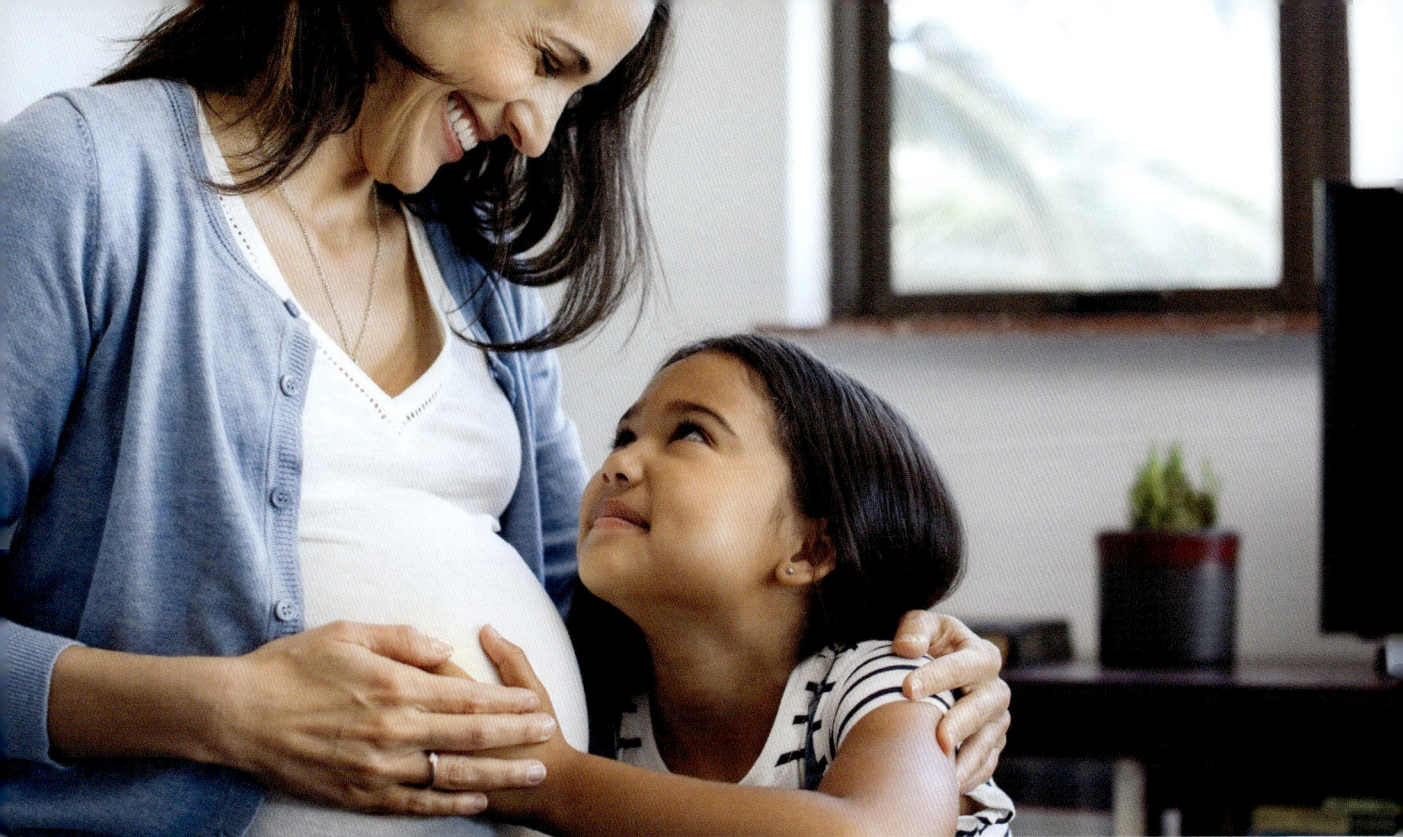

Chapter Two: What Happens During Pregnancy?

"The mother's body is the only environment to which the human infant is adapted."
— **Dr. Donald Winnicott**

When couples are trying to conceive, they often experience a roller coaster of emotions. Being rewarded with one of life's most precious gifts—pregnancy—can change their outlook forever, causing parents-to-be to shift their focus and reevaluate priorities. Pregnancy is a transformative experience, and the divinity of creation is a journey that holds much promise.

In this chapter, we will:

- Discuss how mind, body, and spirit play a crucial role during pregnancy
- Consider common discomforts of pregnancy
- Outline the stages of a baby's growth inside the womb
- Review trends and risks related to vaccination during pregnancy

" *Pregnancy is a transformative experience, and the divinity of creation is a journey that holds much promise.* "

Mind, Body, and Spirit

Mind, body, and spirit are interconnected and play crucial roles throughout the estimated 280 days of pregnancy. Of course, mothers and babies are also connected profoundly after birth.

A mother's thoughts can be as important as the physical care she gives herself and the foods she consumes during pregnancy. Watching a horrific story on the local news may evoke deep empathy but can also elicit a visceral fear response that can cause hypervigilance for days. This is just one example of how uncomfortable thoughts can take over. What a woman feeds her mind shapes her thinking and can directly affect her character and how she interacts with others. What she reads and watches plays a role in overall health and well-being.

Mothers who experience severe psychological stress during pregnancy are at higher risk for prenatal and postpartum complications.[44] Negative thoughts that lead to stress have the ability to suppress the immune system and affect appetite and sleep patterns. Stress is also a known culprit for muscle tension, headaches, and irritability.

Maternal prenatal stress can cause alterations in six different types of hormones (cortisol, glucagon, prolactin, testosterone, estrogen, and progesterone); this can affect both mother and fetus.[45] Studies showing direct effects of stress on babies have identified risks of preterm birth, lower birth weight, alterations in circulatory activity, and neurodevelopmental delays.[46] A baby can feel the "fight or flight" response triggered by the sympathetic nervous system during stressful or traumatic experiences. These experiences do not even have to pose an imminent danger. It might be a heated argument with a friend or partner or a stressful but hard-to-confront situation at work; whatever the situation, the mind keeps spiraling. Thus, cultivating a positive mind-space is an important key to unlocking peace and serenity on the pregnancy journey.

> *Mothers who experience severe psychological stress during pregnancy are at higher risk for prenatal and postpartum complications.*

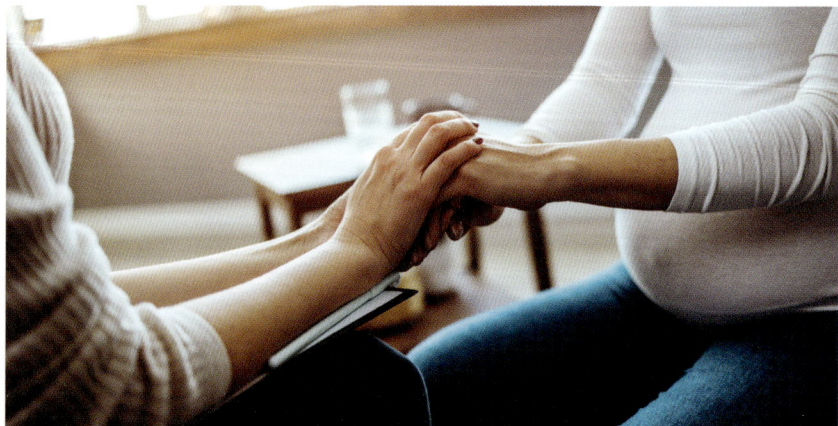

© Dragana hordic/Adobe Stock

Fortunately, there are many ways to develop healthy coping skills to lessen the impacts of fear, anxiety, and stress in everyday life. One example is mindfulness-based practices, which can be helpful in shifting one's mindset. Mindfulness enables individuals to practice sitting with what they are experiencing without judgment or shame. The effects of mindfulness can be life-changing. Everyone is capable of learning mindfulness, though it may take practice to master the skill. Support from a trusted friend, partner, or professional can be helpful.

> "Your baby is in sync with your fear or your happiness. Sing, talk, rub your belly and throw on some soothing music that will help to create connection between you and your baby. You will begin to realize that calm is not too far out of reach."
> — **Thomson et al., Natural Childhood (1995)**

In addition to mindfulness-based practices, other everyday strategies for coping with stress during pregnancy include getting enough sleep, exercising, eating a wholesome diet, and making the most of social support.[47] Paying close attention to feelings and whether there is a sense of lightness and ease can help each woman learn what works best for her.

Spirituality is an important component of well-being. Childbearing is the ideal time to enrich spirituality and understand the spiritual dimensions of childbirth.[48] This is true whether a woman comes to the pregnancy journey already deeply rooted in faith or without previously having had the opportunity to sift through what spirituality means to her.

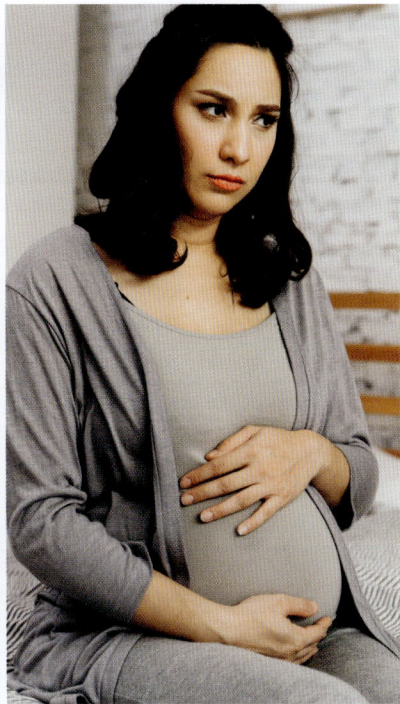

© twinsterphoto/Adobe Stock

> **Childbearing is the ideal time to enrich spirituality and understand the spiritual dimensions of childbirth.**

In the previous chapter, we discussed the importance of eating a nutrient-dense diet from conception through pregnancy and also thereafter. A diet that emphasizes organic grass-fed meats (including organ meats and bone broths), cold-water fish, pastured eggs, high-quality dairy, fruits and vegetables, and properly prepared (soaked, sprouted, or fermented) whole grains—and one that limits or eliminates fast foods, processed foods, and refined sugars—will help keep the body fueled for mother and fetus and may reduce birth complications.

Accessing organic foods can sometimes be challenging. Resources that can facilitate access include coupons, farmers' markets, mail-order companies that specialize in organically raised foods, and community-supported agriculture (CSA) groups. CSAs consist of a community of individuals who pledge support to a farm operation, with the growers and consumers providing mutual support and sharing the risks and benefits of food production. The Weston A. Price Foundation's network of local chapters is a helpful resource for finding local sources and small-scale producers of nutrient-dense foods.[49]

Everyone's financial circumstances are unique, and those circumstances can either improve access or create barriers to healthy nutrition. Fortunately, there are organizations and food programs that can provide assistance to those who need support.

Common Discomforts During Pregnancy

During pregnancy, the baby will grow rapidly, going from a zygote that is the size of a poppy seed to its final weight at birth (see "A Baby's Passage to Earth" on page 22).

The mother may or may not experience varying degrees of discomfort, such as morning sickness, fatigue, heartburn, indigestion, backaches, or stretch marks. What follow are some common discomforts and suggestions about when it may be necessary to seek professional medical advice.

> *During pregnancy, the baby will grow rapidly, going from a zygote that is the size of a poppy seed to its final weight at birth.*

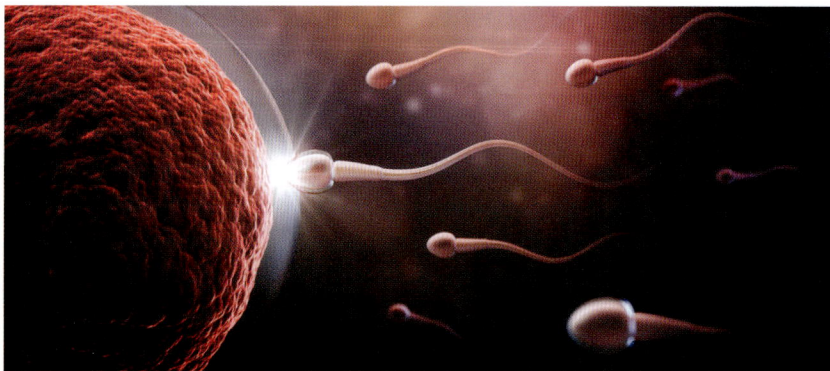

© Anusorn/Adobe Stock

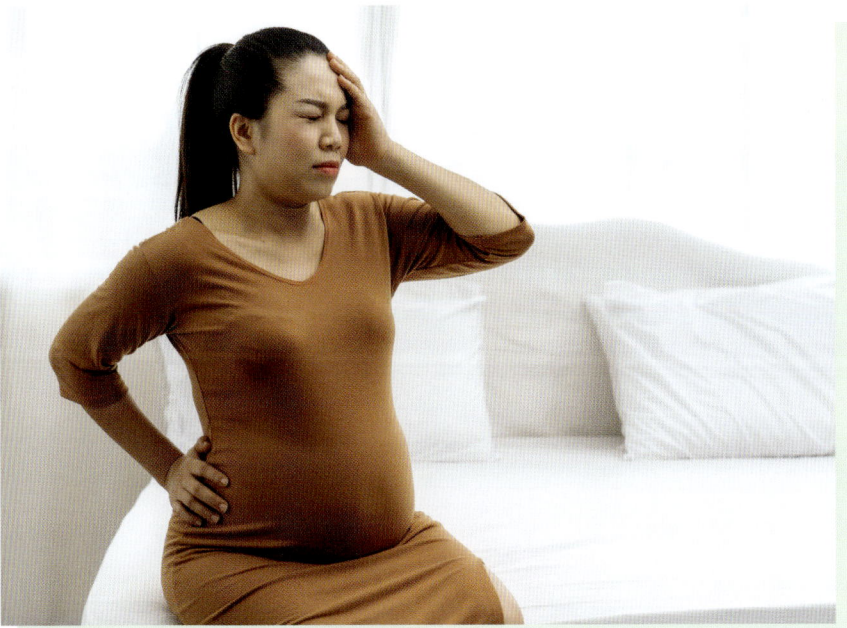

> *Women can prevent or reduce heartburn and indigestion by eating smaller meals throughout the day and avoiding lying down shortly after eating.*

Nausea and Vomiting

Around 50% of all childbearing women experience nausea and sometimes vomiting in the first trimester. Some women have nausea and vomiting throughout pregnancy. These symptoms are due to changes in hormone levels during pregnancy. Factors that may make them worse include stress, traveling, and spicy or fatty foods. Eating smaller meals throughout the day is a proven strategy to mitigate the severity of symptoms. Protein- and gelatin-rich bone broth and chicken broth can help to heal the lining of the stomach.

For some pregnant women, vomiting can be severe, a condition known as hyperemesis gravidarum. This can lead to dehydration and even hospitalization. Communicate with a medical provider or midwife if these symptoms are present.

Heartburn and Indigestion

Both of these symptoms are also very common, especially in the second and third trimesters, caused by pressure on the intestines and stomach (which, in turn, pushes the stomach contents back up into the esophagus). Women can prevent or reduce heartburn and indigestion by eating smaller meals throughout the day and avoiding lying down shortly after eating.

Fatigue

Fatigue can be common during pregnancy as the body is working hard to establish a nourishing environment for the baby. During the first trimester, a feeling of drowsiness may be present throughout the day. The body needs to adjust blood volume and other fluids to account for the growing baby. It is important to pay attention to this fatigue as it can be related to low iron, which is responsible for the oxygen-carrying capacity of red blood cells. Low iron levels result in anemia. A hemoglobin blood test can screen for anemia.

Hemorrhoids

During pregnancy, increased pressure in the rectum and perineum can lead to constipation. Hemorrhoids usually arise later in pregnancy and can be caused by straining during bowel movements. It is important to ensure that the mother consumes an adequate intake of high-fiber foods, including complex carbohydrates, properly prepared whole grains, fruits, and vegetables. Increasing fluid intake and taking supplemental magnesium citrate can also be beneficial.

Swelling or Fluid Retention

Mild swelling is common during pregnancy, but severe swelling that lasts may be a sign of preeclampsia, which is an abnormal condition marked by high blood pressure. Lying on the left side, elevating the legs, and wearing support hose and comfortable shoes may help to relieve swelling. Notify a medical provider or midwife if there is sudden swelling, especially in the hands or face, or if there is rapid weight gain.

Skin Changes

Brown, blotchy patches on the face, forehead, and/or cheeks may appear due to fluctuations in the hormones that stimulate pigmentation of the skin. This is called the mask of pregnancy or chloasma. It often disappears soon after delivery.

Pigmentation may also increase in the skin surrounding the nipples, called the areola. In addition, a dark line often appears down the middle of the stomach. Freckles may darken and moles may grow.

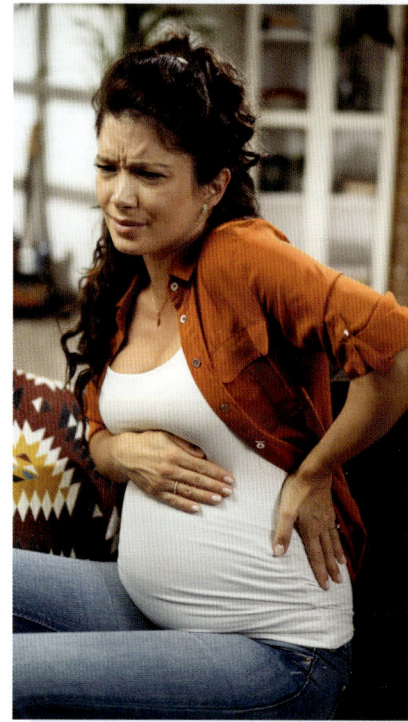

© Just Life/Adobe Stock

> " The body needs to adjust blood volume and other fluids to account for the growing baby. "

Although some health care practitioners recommend using sunscreen when outside to reduce the amount of skin darkening, most sunscreens—even products billed as "safe"—feature endocrine-disrupting and other toxic ingredients (including homosalate, octinoxate, octisalate, avobenzone, oxybenzone, and micro- and nanosize zinc oxide and titanium dioxide) that everyone, including pregnant women and small children, would do well to avoid.[50] Fortunately, coconut oil, a diet high in antioxidants, and protective clothing offer healthy alternatives to sunscreen.[51]

Headaches

Hormonal changes can cause headaches, especially during the first trimester. Rest, proper nutrition, and adequate fluid intake may help ease headache symptoms. Talk with a health care provider or midwife before taking any medicine for this condition. Research associates excessive use of acetaminophen with an increased risk of autism and other adverse outcomes in babies.[52] If a mother experiences a severe headache or a headache that does not resolve, she should contact a healthcare provider, as it may be a sign of preeclampsia.

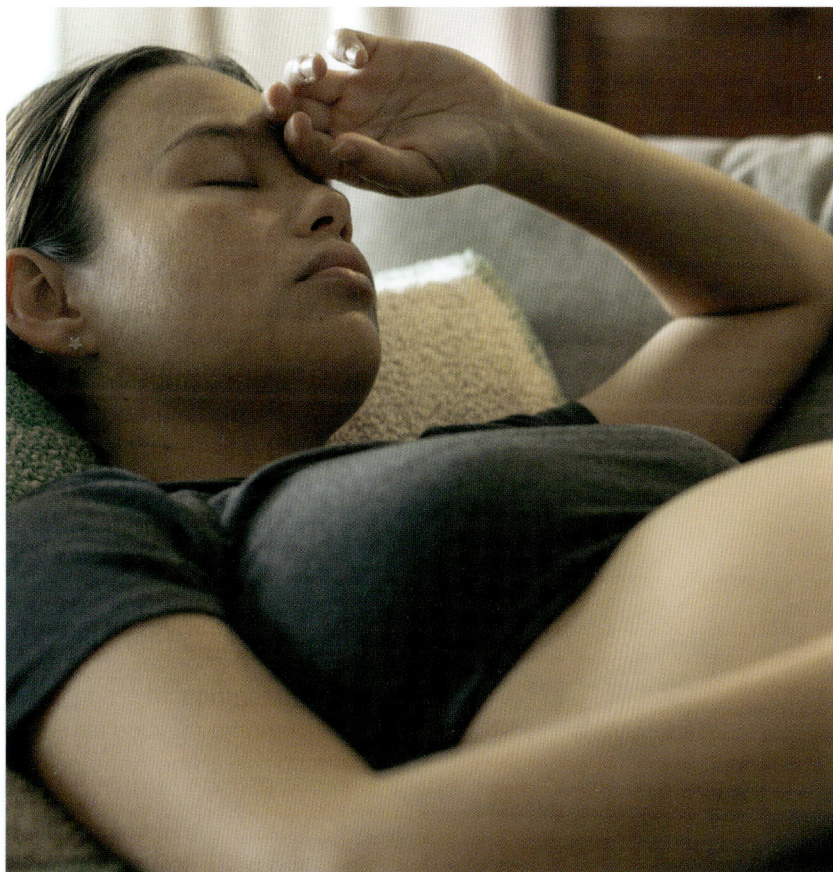

© global moments/Adobe Stock

Back Strain

As a woman's weight increases during pregnancy, her balance changes and her center of gravity is pulled forward, straining her back. Pelvic joints may begin to loosen in preparation for childbirth. Proper posture and proper lifting techniques throughout pregnancy can help reduce back strain.

> " *Hormonal changes can cause headaches, especially during the first trimester.* "

A Baby's Passage to Earth

A fertilized egg (known as a zygote) is the size of a poppy seed. Replicating rapidly, it makes its way down the fallopian tube to the uterus, where it implants as a blastocyst in the uterine lining about a week to ten days after **conception**.

Around the **fourth week**, cells replicate at a rate of one million per second. This ultimately divides into the fetus and the placenta. Note: Because clinicians count pregnancy from the first day of the last menstrual period, "four weeks" is usually only two weeks post-conception and about one week after implantation; for women with erratic menstrual cycles, pregnancy dating can sometimes be significantly "off."

During the **second month**, the fetus is the size of a raspberry. The heart starts to beat, and the brain grows 100,000 cells per minute. The fetus is now 10,000 times bigger than at conception.

During the **third month**, the fetus is the size of a lemon. At this time, the womb is a sensory playground. The fetus can now move hands, suck fingers, smile, and hear mom's voice and heartbeat. Toxins from tobacco, vaping, or marijuana smoke can have harmful effects on the developing fetus and may actually cause the fetus to cringe.

During the **fourth month** of pregnancy, the fetus is the approximate size of a tomato. The head is half the size of the whole body. Taste buds have started to develop, and fetal programming begins to take place. A fetus learns to appreciate different tastes when the mother eats a variety of different foods. (This can help a child become a less fussy eater later in life.)

During the **fifth month** of pregnancy, the fetus is the size of a dragon fruit. This stage kick-starts a steep growth spurt. The teeth, hair, eyebrows, and eyelashes all develop around this time. The mother's voice becomes clearer. If mom has not already felt her baby wriggle or kick, she will soon! Her baby quickly learns that for every action, there is a reaction. A mother can rub her belly when she feels her baby kick, letting baby know, with a soft voice, that she is present.

During the **sixth month** of pregnancy, the fetus is the size of a small cauliflower. This is the time when a baby can start to learn to communicate. The baby's eyes may open, and simple facial expressions will begin. The cerebral cortex of the brain splits into two hemispheres at this time. Believe it or not, the baby only sees a blur but can respond to light.

During the **seventh month**, the fetus is the size of a pineapple.

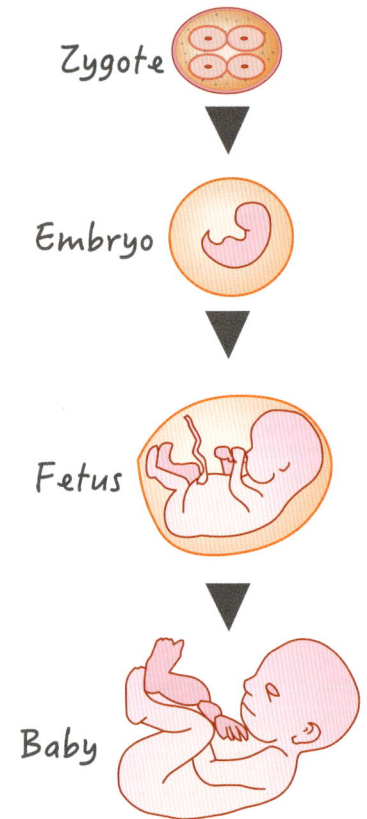

Zygote

Embryo

Fetus

Baby

© Lucky Soul/Adobe Stock

> " *Around the fourth week, cells replicate at a rate of one million per second. This ultimately divides into the fetus and the placenta.* "

The sleep and wake cycle is developing. The hair is visible. The baby is now even more aware of the mother's voice and language and can respond with an increased heart rate and movements. Teeth will have formed under the gums.

During the **eighth month**, the fetus is the size of a small melon. The brain is now functional, and the baby spends most of the time in a sleep state. The lungs are almost fully formed, and the baby has already practiced breathing by inhaling amniotic fluid. The nervous system is ready! However, the baby's immune system is still immature. Bodyguards from the mother's system will protect the baby well into infancy.

When the fetus officially enters the **ninth month** of the journey, the baby will be the size of a jackfruit. At this point, babies have coordinated reflexes and can close and blink their eyes, turn their heads, and grasp firmly, as well as respond to light, touch, and sounds.

Month 10, which encompasses weeks 37 to 40, is the final month. Babies are preparing for their debut on Earth. There may be less movement as the womb becomes tighter and the baby's position changes to prepare for birth. Ideally, the baby's head should be face down in the uterus.

> *During the seventh month, the fetus is the size of a pineapple.*

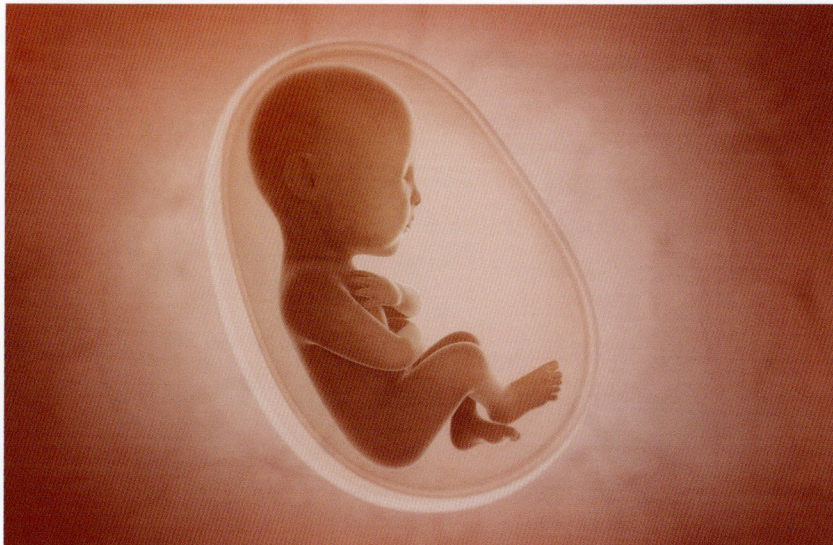

© adimas/Adobe Stock

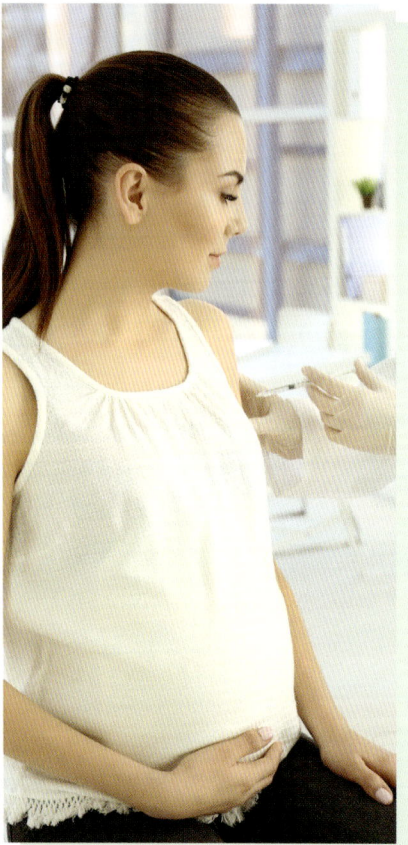
© Africa Studio/Adobe Stock

Vaccination During Pregnancy

Many women instinctively know that pregnancy is a time to be cautious about medications. A 2018 study showed that pregnant women's top concern about taking medications during pregnancy had to do with the drugs' potential impact on fetal development.[53]

Medical history validates women's innate caution and indicates that they cannot always count on healthcare providers and regulators to prioritize developmental safety. For example, for two of the 20th century's most infamous developmental toxicity disasters,[54] the Food and Drug Administration (FDA) turned a blind eye for years or decades before halting them. Though the FDA never approved the late-1950s drug thalidomide, the agency allowed over 2.5 million doses to be administered to 20,000 pregnant women under cover of "clinical trials"; afterwards, the FDA acknowledged serious birth defects in just 17 babies—a figure hotly disputed by U.S. thalidomide victims—later admitting that the drug had adversely impacted "thousands of children" worldwide.[55] Meanwhile, the FDA approved diethylstilbestrol (DES) in 1947 but waited until 1971 to issue a soft-pedaled warning to pregnant women; DES caused multigenerational effects that persist to this day.

> " Medical history validates women's innate caution and indicates that they cannot always count on healthcare providers and regulators to prioritize developmental safety. "

Industry and regulators like to dismiss these incidents as ancient history, but modern medical websites for the public continue to furnish long lists of drugs with birth defect risks equal to or greater than thalidomide, including widely prescribed drugs for acne, hypertension, and depression.[56] These same sites also describe heavy metals such as lead and mercury as known developmental toxins, yet they tell women that flu shots (some of which contain mercury) are completely safe "any time during … pregnancy." Toxicologists warn that mercury toxicity is time-dependent as well as dose-dependent and that even tiny doses "may cause extensive adverse effects later in life."[57]

Why, then, does the Centers for Disease Control and Prevention (CDC) recommend vaccines for pregnant women, beginning with flu shots? Until around 2006, doctors and pregnant women largely ignored the agency's recommendations, but that changed after the CDC stepped up its aggressive promotion of pregnancy flu shots. In 2011, CDC and medical trade organizations additionally began recommending that pregnant women get the Tdap vaccine (tetanus-diphtheria-acellular pertussis),[58] which, among other ingredients, contains neurotoxic aluminum.[59] Following the 2011 recommendation, Tdap coverage in pregnancy increased substantially.[60] By April 2020, three out of five pregnant women (61%) were receiving flu shots, and nearly that many (57%) were getting Tdap vaccines.[61]

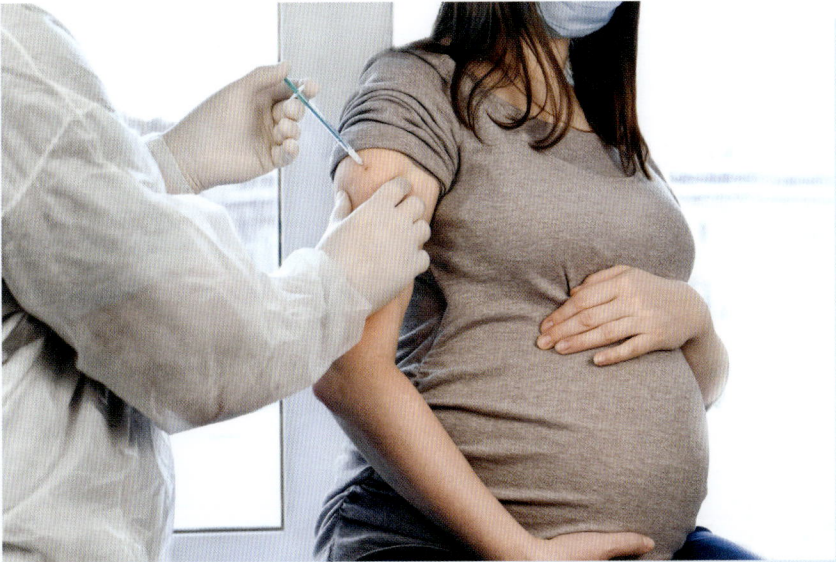

© Marina Demidiuk/Adobe Stock

*By April 2020, **three out of five pregnant women (61%) were receiving flu shots, and nearly that many (57%) were getting Tdap vaccines.***

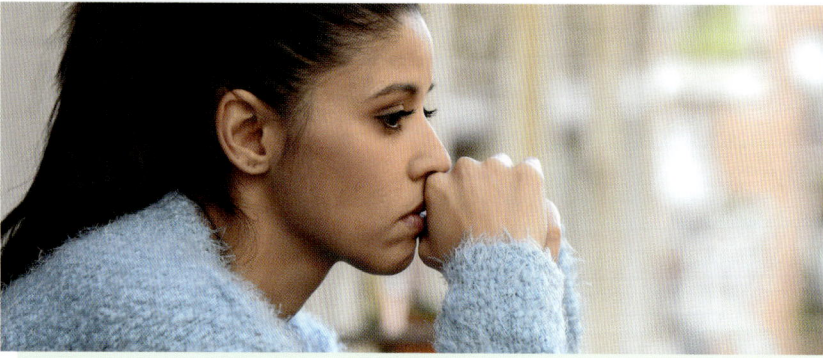

© Wordley Calvo Stock/Adobe Stock

Proponents of maternal vaccination sometimes pay lip service to the need for an extra-high evidentiary bar for pregnancy vaccines—stating that they "must provide efficacy in decreasing morbidity for the pregnant woman, her fetus, and the neonate" and "demonstrate safety or lack of evidence of harm"[62]—but the actual evidence base is flimsy. As its 2006 proof of flu shot safety during pregnancy, for example, CDC pointed to a grand total of two retrospective epidemiological studies of medical records—one published in 1973.[63] No prelicensure studies of Tdap safety during pregnancy were available when the CDC later recommended maternal Tdap shots. An archived package insert for one Tdap brand admitted, "It is also not known whether Adacel vaccine can cause fetal harm when administered to a pregnant woman or can affect reproduction capacity."[64] The insert now omits that statement.[65]

The World Health Organization (WHO), in 2013, acknowledged "the limited amount of clinical trial data on pregnant women,"[66] though a year earlier it had published a position paper identifying pregnant women "as the highest priority group for countries considering initiation or expansion of programmes for seasonal influenza vaccination."[67] The FDA's Center for Biologics Evaluation and Research (CBER)—which regulates vaccines and other biologics—says that researchers should assess developmental toxicity in animal models "prior to licensure of vaccines intended for maternal immunization"[68] but admits, "lack of adverse effects on embryo/fetal development in an animal study does not necessarily imply absence of risk for humans."[69] Still, the widely shared default position is that "there is no documented causal evidence of developmental or reproductive toxic effects in humans following the use of [any] approved vaccine."[70]

> " As its 2006 proof of flu shot safety during pregnancy...CDC pointed to a grand total of two retrospective epidemiological studies of medical records. "

26

Published reports point in the opposite direction, suggesting an increased risk of miscarriages and elevated risks of birth defects and autism in the offspring of mothers who received influenza vaccines during pregnancy (as described by Children's Health Defense in multiple articles).[71,72,73] Although Tdap evidence is still emerging, the WHO's global VigiBase database (which currently collects reports of drug- and vaccine-related adverse events from 150 countries) provides some clues.[74] A search of the database's public-facing platform, VigiAccess,[75] indicates that over two-thirds (68%) of all adverse events reported to VigiBase for vaccines containing diphtheria, tetanus, and pertussis active ingredients have occurred since 2010, half (49%) have been in women, and 8% have been in the 18–44-year age group. Moreover, the flu and Tdap shots have never resulted in any statistically significant reduction in the outcomes they are supposed to influence.[76,77]

In addition to influenza and Tdap vaccines, the CDC also recommends:

- COVID-19 shots for all pregnant women, as well as lactating women and women who are trying to get pregnant (or who "might become pregnant in the future")[78]
- Five vaccines—hepatitis A and B, meningococcal vaccines (ACWY or B), polio—depending on the pregnant woman's "circumstances," or based on "risk vs. benefit," or "if otherwise indicated" or "if needed"[79]
- Five potential travel vaccines

For several other vaccines, the CDC takes no position one way or another. In fact, there are only four vaccines—human papillomavirus (HPV), live influenza, measles-mumps-rubella (MMR), and varicella (chickenpox)—that the agency does not recommend for pregnant women at all.[80] Meanwhile, many more pregnancy vaccines are in the pipeline.[81]

> *There are only four vaccines...that the agency does not recommend for pregnant women at all. Meanwhile, many more pregnancy vaccines are in the pipeline.*

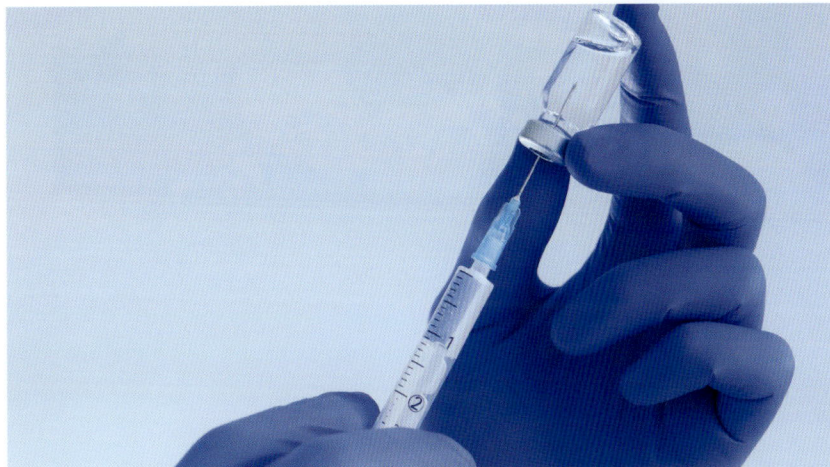

A 2017 assessment of titanium dioxide nanoparticles—a modern product included in many cosmetics and drugs—warned of the significant and potentially devastating effects of nanoparticle exposure on "millions of pregnant mothers and their offspring,"[82] but there have been no comparable studies or warnings for nanoparticle-containing vaccines. In fact, lipid nanoparticles (LNPs)[83] are key components of the Pfizer and Moderna COVID-19 shots that the CDC continues to urge on pregnant women, despite evidence that the LNPs are "highly inflammatory," lethal in animal models, and, in some scientists' view, tantamount to "poison."[84] Increasingly, other vaccines also contain nanoparticulate ingredients (some intended and some not).[85,86]

Medical experts have tried to sound the alarm about the COVID-19 shots' impacts on pregnant women and their babies.

- One American OB-GYN described an "off-the-charts" rise in sudden fetal death[87]—"way, way beyond" what the CDC ordinarily would consider a safety signal—as well as other adverse fetal outcomes (such as fetal malformation and fetal cardiac arrest) and significantly increased rates of miscarriage and menstrual abnormalities.[88]

- In October 2022, a Florida-based OB-GYN shared observations on social media about a 50% decrease in new OB patients (suggesting infertility) and a 50% increased miscarriage rate in her practice, as well as substantial increases in abnormal pap smears and cervical malignancies.[89]

- Around the same time, the Scottish government ordered an investigation into the "spike in newborn baby deaths" in 2021 and 2022—describing the increase as "larger than expected from chance alone."[90,91]

The bottom line, as available data show, is that none of the vaccines promoted for pregnant women are safe for babies or their moms.[92]

> *None of the vaccines promoted for pregnant women are safe for babies or their moms.*

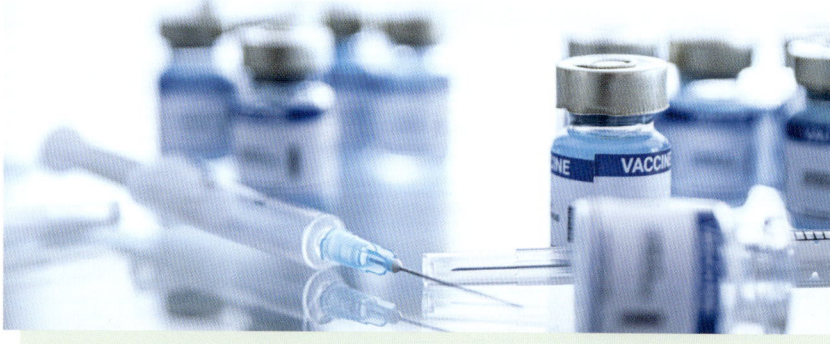

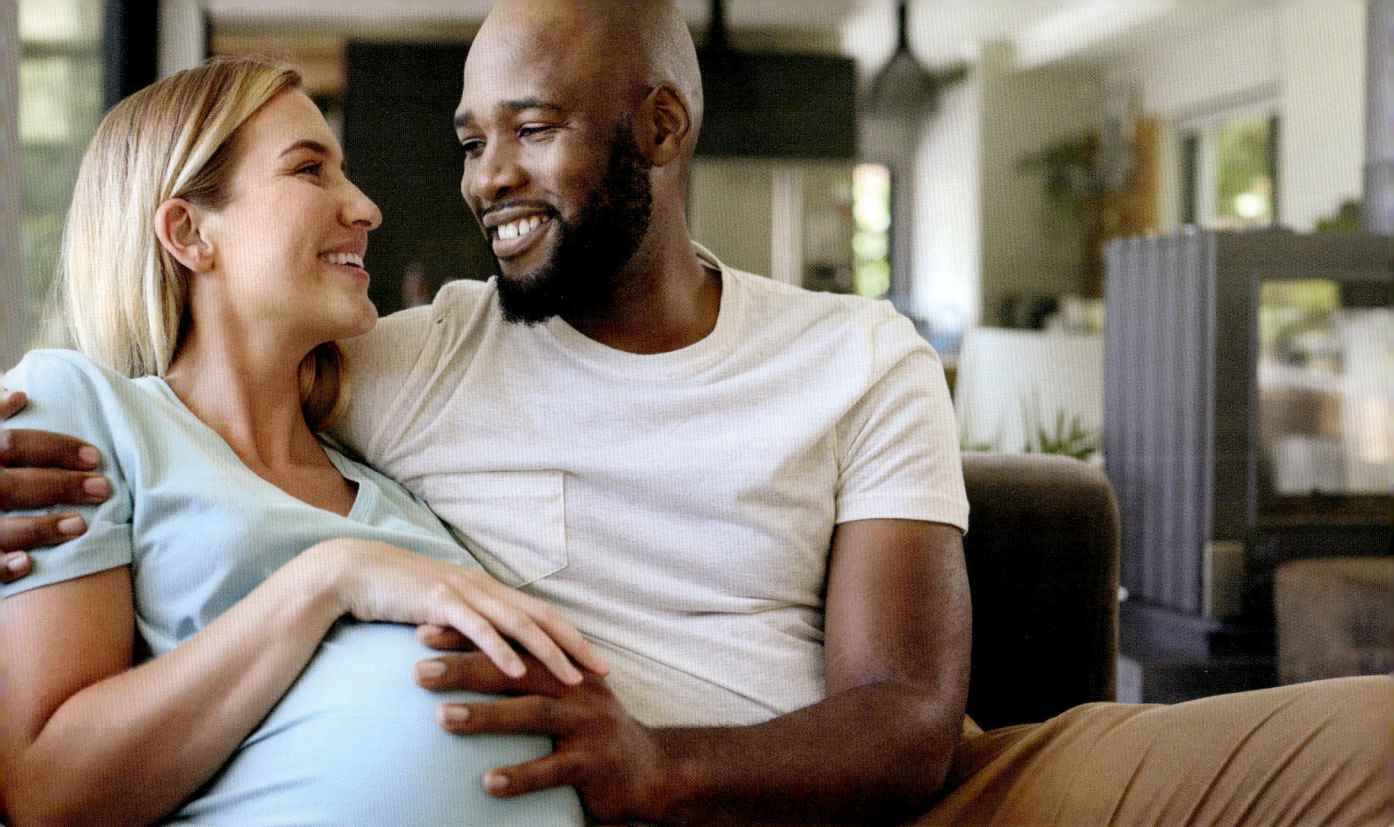

Chapter Three: Planning for Childbirth

"The power of the birth plan is not the actual plan, it's the process of being educated about all your options."
— **Jen McLellan, Plus Size Birth**

Many believe that the awesome responsibility of parenting begins after new parents take their baby home from the hospital. However, many important decisions affecting the health and vitality of the baby begin long before that. The choices parents make throughout a pregnancy can affect the baby's future well-being.

This includes the choice of obstetrician, midwife, doula, or other individuals to support the mother during childbirth, and the choices parents make about day-of-birth medical interventions.

> **The choices parents make throughout a pregnancy can affect the baby's future well-being.**

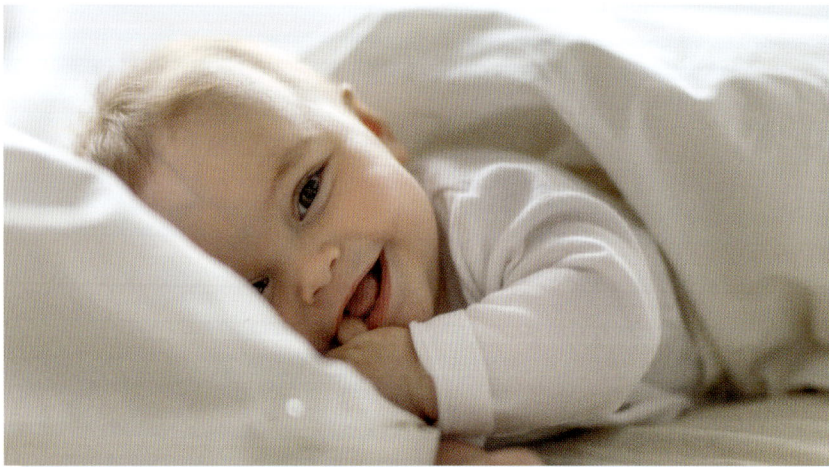
© Louis-Paul Photo/Adobe Stock

> *There are certain questions that women should ask when choosing healthcare providers who will become intimate members of a birth team.*

In this chapter, we will:

- Provide guidance and resources to help parents understand the differences and similarities between hospital births, home births, and birth centers

- Encourage parents to develop a birth plan that reflects their preferences as to what is safest for mother and baby

- Review the risks of day-of-birth vitamin K shots and hepatitis B vaccination

Exploring Childbirth Options

Many parents place a lot of trust in the health care providers who specialize in childbirth and rely on providers to help them develop an individualized plan. Unfortunately, the average obstetrician is unlikely to ask a mother what she wants. If the provider does ask, that person is probably a good choice!

Couples who are embarking on the journey of parenthood deserve to have a birth plan that leaves them feeling empowered and fully informed about all the options available to them so they can make sound decisions weighing the risks and benefits of each option.

There are certain questions that women should ask when choosing healthcare providers who will become intimate members of a birth team (see "10 Questions to Ask When Preparing for Childbirth"). Answers to these fundamental questions will help a mother get to know the provider and evaluate whether they are suitable for her needs.[93] Women or couples can ask these questions at the initial prenatal consultation or the next prenatal visit. This information can help parents-to-be to make the best decision for themselves and their baby.

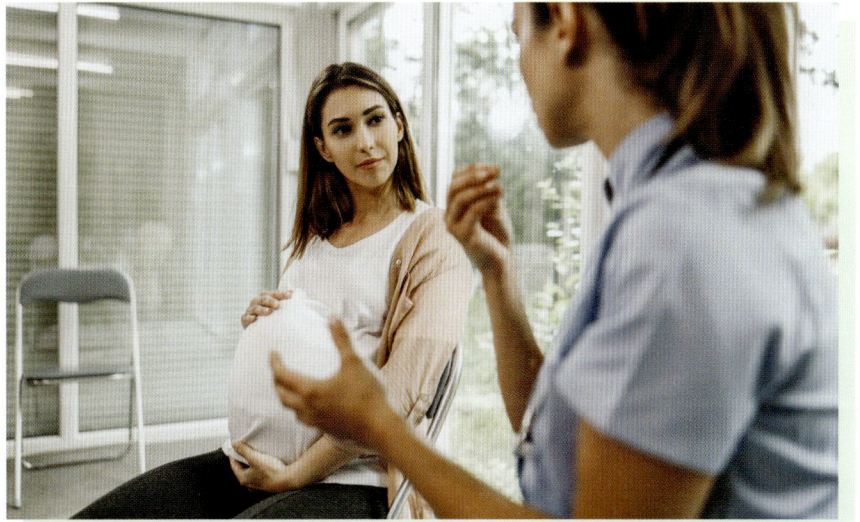

© milanmarkovic78/Adobe Stock

The Rise of Hospital Births

It hasn't been that long since it was common for midwives to deliver infants in the comfort of the family's own home. Although most of North America and Europe had public and private hospital systems by the mid-1800s, having a baby in a hospital did not become common until the early 1900s.[94] The change occurred during the industrial age when dirty and cramped living quarters made it more difficult for women to give birth at home safely. This concern precipitated the first birthing hospitals. However, affluent women continued to have their babies at home.

> *Although most of North America and Europe had public and private hospital systems by the mid-1800s, having a baby in a hospital did not become common until the early 1900s.*

In 1914, Boston opened one of the developed world's first maternity (baby) hospitals for all income classes. By the 1920s, advances in medical technology had led to the practice of minimizing labor pain with morphine and scopolamine, which providers used to induce an amnesic, semi-conscious state that eventually became known as "Twilight Sleep." The popularity of Twilight Sleep and propaganda promoting hospitals as the safest and most sanitary places to give birth led to the majority of babies being born in hospitals by the end of the 1930s, with hospital birth perceived as ideal by the 1940s.

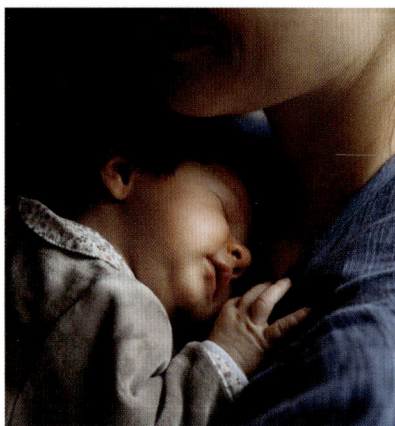

© RFBSIP/Adobe Stock

Hospital Birth Today

Today, the majority of women in developed countries have their babies in hospitals. Some countries' professional obstetric organizations actively discourage home births. Having a baby in a hospital means there will probably be a higher level of care, more pain management options, and healthcare providers present in case of an emergency. Hospital births also offer more medical technology, anesthetics, surgical procedures, and postnatal emergent care. However, for low-risk women in particular, these technical advances are not without risks such as excess cesarean deliveries ("C-sections"). As birth options expert Henci Goer has observed, "We have abundant evidence of the gross overuse of tests, drugs, restrictions, and procedures in hospitals, the toll of its consequent harms, and the low use of practices known to promote healthy, physiologic birth."[95]

> *Today, the majority of women in developed countries have their babies in hospitals.*

Parents-to-be should know that COVID-19 had a significant impact on hospital birthing practices, and many hospitals have retained some or all of the new protocols put in place, such as masking, testing, limiting the number of support persons allowed, and separating newborns from their mothers.[96] A New York study of women who had hospital births during the height of the pandemic found that the women experienced lower birth satisfaction along with more postpartum anxiety, stress, and depression, including "birth-related PTSD."[97]

If parents and providers deem a hospital birth the best decision, the obstetrician should provide full transparency for all medications and procedures that the hospital staff will offer. The provider should be able to address all of the following prior to delivery:

1. The names of the drugs, procedures, or other interventions likely to be proposed

2. The reasons (benefits) for proposing the drugs, procedures, or interventions

3. The potential risks of the proposed drugs, procedures, or interventions

4. Ramifications if the proposed drugs, procedures, or interventions are not used, or if there is an extended wait period before using them

5. Alternatives to the proposed drugs, procedures, or interventions

6. Restrictions or other policies related to COVID-19

There are circumstances where hospital birth may seem preferable. For example, women who have a known prenatal risk factor such as preeclampsia or an underlying health condition such as diabetes or high blood pressure may opt to give birth in a hospital setting where advanced support is readily available, since these conditions may place a mother at increased risk for prenatal and postpartum complications. These types of concerns can warrant access to technology to closely monitor mother and child.

If a woman has experienced preterm labor in the past and is at risk for preterm labor again, this, too, might point to a hospital birth plan. If the fetus has a prenatal diagnosis that places the fetus at higher risk, an expert team of providers should be available after the birth.

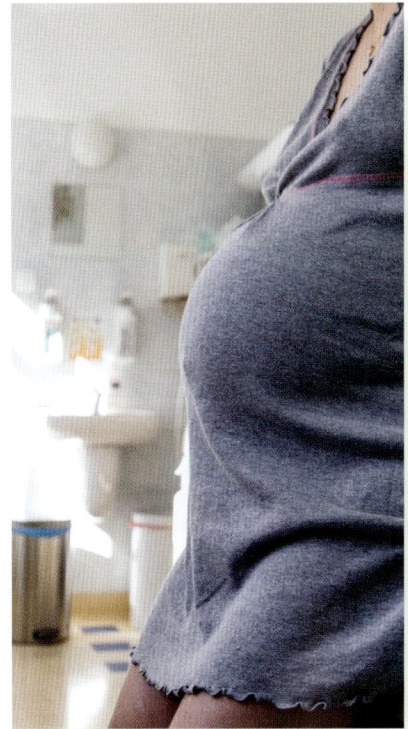
© mathom/Adobe Stock

> *If a woman has experienced preterm labor in the past and is at risk for preterm labor again, this, too, might point to a hospital birth plan.*

In the U.S., the cost of an uncomplicated vaginal birth varies from hospital to hospital, ranging from a few thousand dollars to over $30,000; more often than not, it comes with a hefty price tag. According to the nonprofit organization FAIR Health, the national average for a vaginal delivery is $12,290, and the national average for a C-section is $16,907 (without insurance).[98] That's 40% and 60% higher, respectively, than in Switzerland, the next most expensive country. In 2014, researchers at the University of California, San Francisco, found that in California, an uncomplicated vaginal birth could cost up to $37,227, depending on the hospital.[99] The study showed that C-sections ranged from $8,312 to almost $71,000.

Insurance coverage for childbirth varies widely, depending on the details of a particular plan and the individual insurance company's interpretation of what it should cover. Expectant mothers should speak to their insurance company and ask for the itemized estimated costs for a vaginal and cesarean delivery based on their hospital (or birth center) of choice.

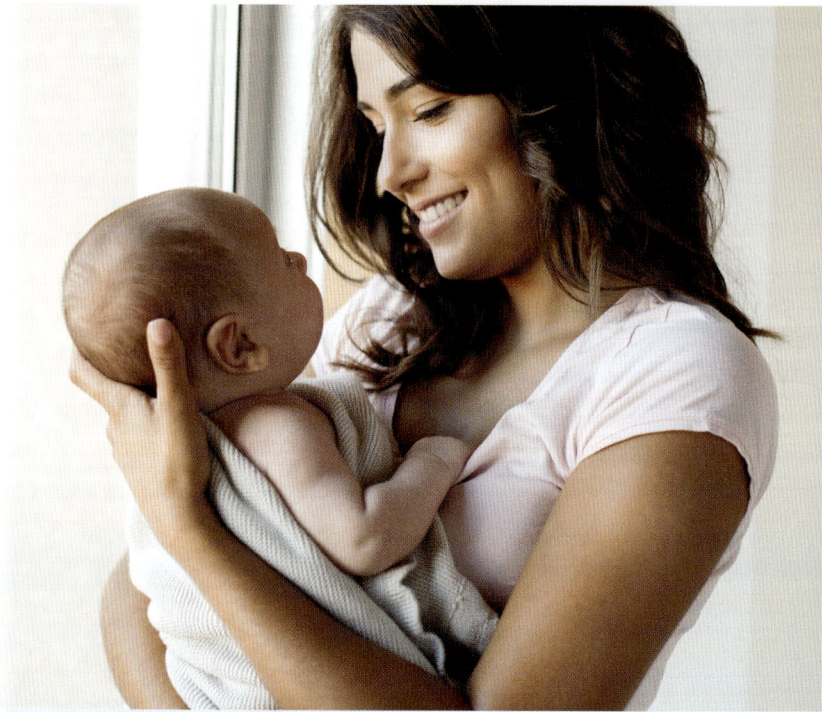

© Trendsetter Images/Adobe Stock

When having a baby at a hospital, it is a good idea to ensure good communication with the obstetrician. Because delivering a baby in a hospital setting can elicit anxiety and feel unfamiliar and restrictive, it can be wise to pack a bag of clothes (including some cherished comfort measures) and enlist a support professional such as a doula,[100] or involve a trusted friend or family member who is willing to offer support during delivery. However, there may be limitations on how many support individuals a hospital will allow to be present during delivery.

> 66
> *In the U.S., the cost of an uncomplicated vaginal birth varies from hospital to hospital, ranging from a few thousand dollars to over $30,000.*
> 99

Home Birth

For centuries, women delivered children in the comfort of their own homes, and there was little interference with the natural progression of giving birth. Today in the United States, however, only 35,000 births per year occur in the home, representing just 0.9% of all births.[101] An estimated one-fourth of home births are unplanned or unattended. Since 2020, restrictions related to COVID-19 have prompted a growing number of women to turn to home birth.[102]

Home birth allows for greater privacy and offers mothers more choices about who may accompany them during the birth process as well as different pain management approaches. For some women who are preparing to deliver, the pain experienced during childbirth can seem scary; having a home birth allows for the use of nonpharmacologic remedies to mitigate pain during labor[103] but limits access to the more invasive pain management interventions that hospitals typically use.[104]

Each woman has the right to make a medically informed decision regarding how she chooses to give birth. When considering a home birth, it is crucial that a mother understand both the risks and benefits of home birth and seek guidance from a trusted provider.[105] Most importantly, home birth providers should inform women about factors critical to reducing perinatal mortality rates and achieving favorable home birth outcomes. These factors include:

- The selection of appropriate home birth candidates
- The availability of a certified nurse-midwife, whose education and licensure meet International Confederation of Midwives' Global Standards for Midwifery Education, or a physician practicing obstetrics within an integrated and regulated health system
- Ready access to consultation
- Access to safe and timely transport to a nearby hospital in case of need

> *Today in the United States...only 35,000 births per year occur in the home, representing just 0.9% of all births.*

© Miramiska/Adobe Stock

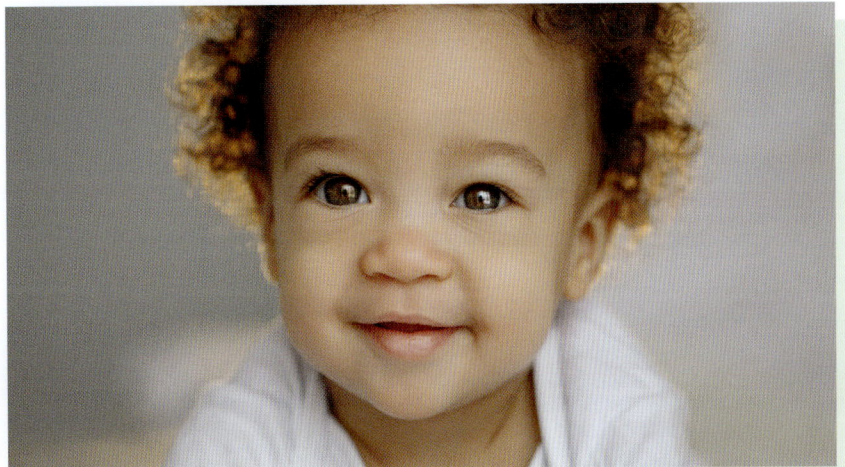

The substantial literature addressing home birth safety generally reports that for low-risk mothers in the care of credentialed midwives, the safety of planned home births is comparable to that in birth centers and hospitals.

Based on a nationwide study conducted in 2021, the estimated average cost of a home birth in the United States is $4,650, which is significantly below existing cost estimates for an uncomplicated birth center or hospital birth. The study indicated that "each shift of one percent of births from hospitals to homes would represent an annual cost savings" of at least $321 million.[106]

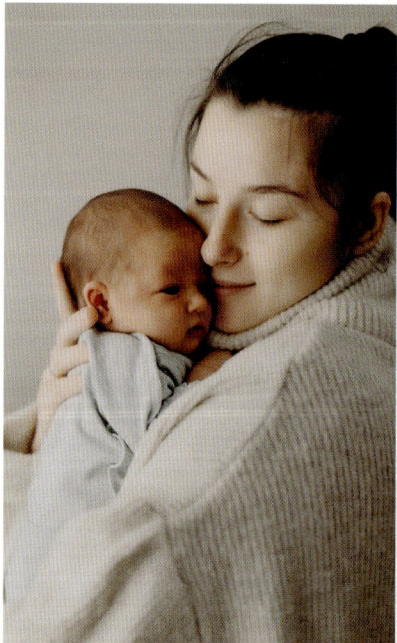

© Ananass/Adobe Stock

Birth Centers

With less than one percent of women choosing home birth, 99% of women continue to opt for a dedicated space for giving birth. Freestanding birth centers are an alternative to the hospital setting and have become quite popular.[107] In contrast to hospitals, freestanding birth centers offer a more home-like approach. Although designed to provide a non-medical setting for birth, freestanding birth facilities generally have partnerships with nearby hospitals and doctors in the event that a woman requires more specialized care.

Stand-alone centers focus on low-risk pregnancies and births, and typically use a midwifery or wellness model. This means moms-to-be go into labor without being induced, and they receive little-to-no pain medication throughout the process. This is often referred to as natural or unmedicated birth. Compared to hospitals, research indicates that birth centers result in lower rates of preterm and surgical birth, as well as "increased breastfeeding success and overall positive experience of birth."[108]

> *In contrast to hospitals, freestanding birth centers offer a more home-like approach.*

Natural Interventions During Labor and Delivery

No matter what option a woman chooses, there are a number of interventions during labor that can help with natural childbirth.

Lamaze, a method started in Russia,[109] uses distraction during contractions ("psychoprophylaxis") to decrease the perception of pain and thereby reduce discomfort. In a Lamaze class, partners learn controlled deep breathing, massage, concentration, and how to maintain control during labor. There are Lamaze classes all over the country.[110]

There has been an increase in the number of couples who choose water deliveries, with studies confirming their safety.[111] Giving birth in a warm tub of water can help a woman relax, and advocates also believe that water helps the baby enter the world with less light, sound, and dramatic change.[112] The buoyancy also helps to alleviate pressure and discomfort during vaginal delivery. There are some contraindications to water delivery, and childbirth providers do not recommend it for high-risk pregnancies.

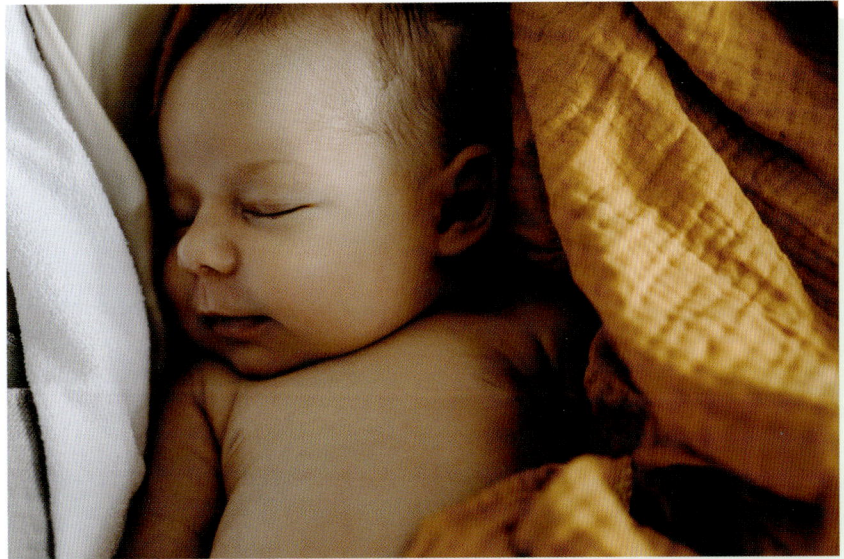

© Boston Natalia/Adobe Stock

The Alexander Technique and the Bradley Method integrate natural interventions,[113,114] including a focus on posture, breathing techniques, and movement, to help mitigate discomfort during labor. Dr. Robert Bradley developed the Bradley Method in the late 1940s to help women deliver naturally, with few or no drugs. Bradley Method courses emphasize excellent nutrition, exercise, relaxation techniques to manage pain and the effective involvement of the husband or partner as a coach.

The Alexander Technique encompasses techniques for sitting, standing, and moving with safety, efficiency, and ease. Anyone, including a pregnant woman, can learn to release muscular tension to increase breathing capacity and restore the body's original poise and proper posture.

> " No matter what option a woman chooses, there are a number of interventions during labor that can help with natural childbirth. "

Support During Childbirth

Women who are nearing the estimated date of their baby's arrival may feel confident that they will be "ready to go" when the baby decides to make his or her debut. However, it is advisable to have backup options. When couples discuss birthing options with their obstetrician or midwife, they should agree on a "Plan B" just in case "Plan A" does not go smoothly.

Communicating closely with one's chosen provider can be essential during the time leading up to a baby's birth. In addition, research shows how helpful it can be to have the continuous presence of an individual who can provide emotional support, comfort measures, advocacy, information, and advice during labor. This individual can be a trained person—such as a doula, midwife, or nurse—or a friend or family member. The presence of a support person leads to improved outcomes that include:

- An increased likelihood of vaginal delivery
- Decreased use of epidurals
- Improved Apgar scores (a five-category scoring system, with a maximum of 10 points, that clinicians use to assess newborns one minute and five minutes after they are born)
- Greater maternal satisfaction

Midwives and doulas are experts in the birthing process. They can assist mothers with education regarding pelvic floor physiotherapy during pregnancy, which may aid as a preventive measure and serve as a way to prepare physically and mentally for labor and delivery. There continues to be strong evidence in favor of pelvic floor muscle training with a physiotherapist to prevent urinary incontinence during pregnancy and after delivery.

> "When couples discuss birthing options with their obstetrician or midwife, they should agree on a "Plan B" just in case "Plan A" does not go smoothly.

© Dragon Images/Adobe Stock

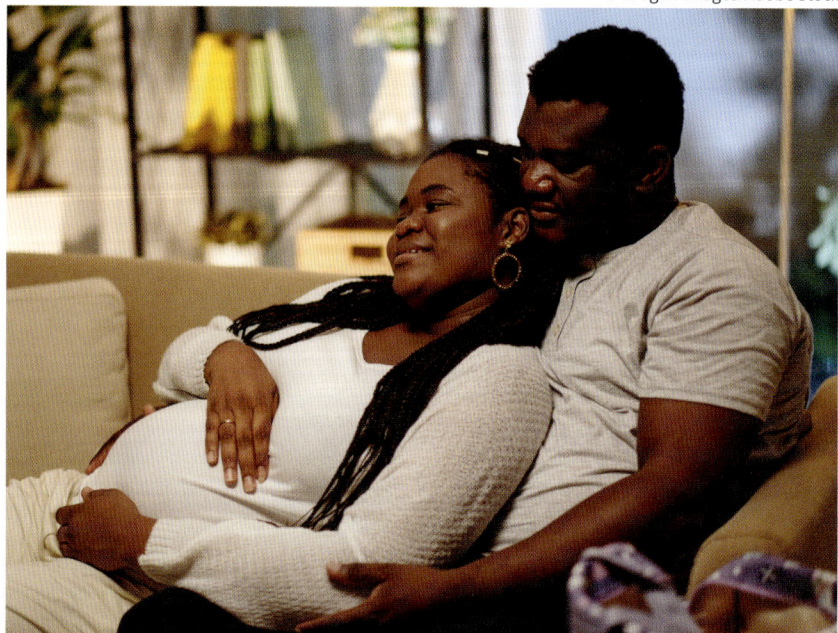

Prenatal massage can help decrease tension and promote relaxation. The massage provider does not have to be a professional; a loved one is capable of this therapeutic touch.

Birthing classes are available in most areas. The content of prenatal classes varies, with some classes focusing on first-time parents' expectations of the birthing process, and others focusing on promoting techniques to prepare mothers physically and emotionally for birth.

Day-of-Birth Medical Interventions

Unless parents specifically refuse, nearly all babies are subject to two medical interventions on the day of birth: vitamin K injections and hepatitis B vaccination.

Vitamin K Injections

The American Academy of Pediatrics (AAP), a medical trade group that frequently helps promote CDC policies, recommends intramuscular injections of synthetic vitamin K (phytonadione) within hours of birth for all newborn infants, including those born prematurely.[115] AAP and CDC promote the injections as protection against rare cases of severe bleeding due to deficiency—risks that are higher when mothers have a history of taking anti-tuberculosis or anti-seizure medications.[116]

© Louis-Paul Photo/Adobe Stock

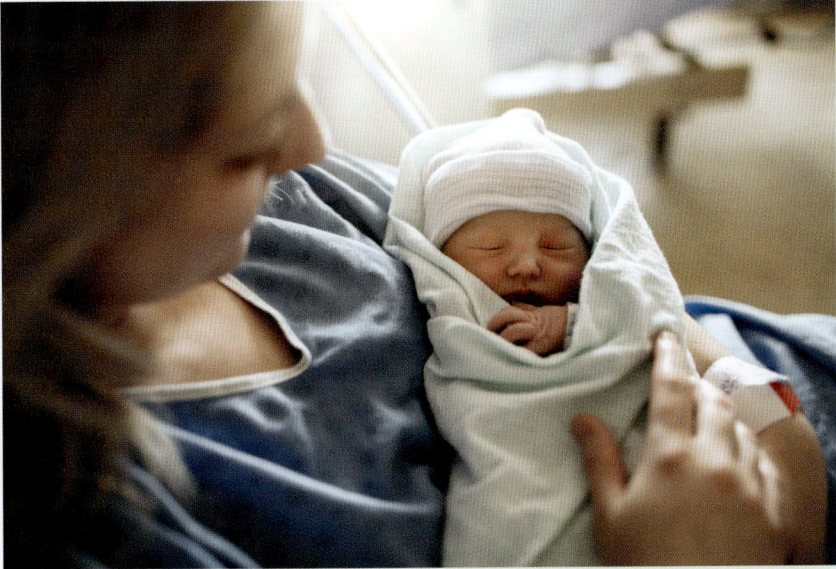

Prenatal massage can help decrease tension and promote relaxation.

The two organizations generally do not tell new parents about:

- The shot's aluminum content (the insert for Pfizer's vitamin K product states, "This product contains aluminum that may be toxic")[117]
- The potential toxicity of the shot's preservative benzyl alcohol (including an association with a fatal "gasping syndrome" in premature infants)[118]
- The risk of fatal hypersensitivity or anaphylactic reactions[119]
- The risk of red blood cell breakdown (hemolysis) and jaundice, especially in preemies
- Other potential adverse reactions such as turning blue, dizziness, rapid and weak pulse, excessive sweating, hypotension, and shortness of breath
- The absence of studies on carcinogenicity or mutagenesis

Alert to these risks and unknowns, more parents than ever before are saying no to vitamin K shots, with a 2020 study describing refusal rates of up to 3.2% in hospital settings and 15% and 31% in home and birth center settings, respectively.[120]

Recent research indicates that synthetic vitamin K shots also work against nature's plan. Babies "are born with levels of vitamin K that are lower than those of adults, for a reason": their digestive system needs to mature to be able to absorb vitamin K.[121] Moreover, leaving the umbilical cord intact after birth, preferably until the cord stops pulsing—a practice called "delayed cord clamping"—allows babies' "inbuilt system [of umbilical stem cells] to protect against and repair damage and bleeding in their organs." Natural vitamin K in breast milk also reaches infants, decreasing the risk of deficiency bleeding.

Hepatitis B Vaccination

Since 1991, the CDC has recommended hepatitis B vaccination for all babies on their first day of life,[122] followed by two more doses in early infancy. Whereas newborns of mothers who do not have hepatitis B have virtually no chance of developing hepatitis B illness, the vaccines impose significant risks.

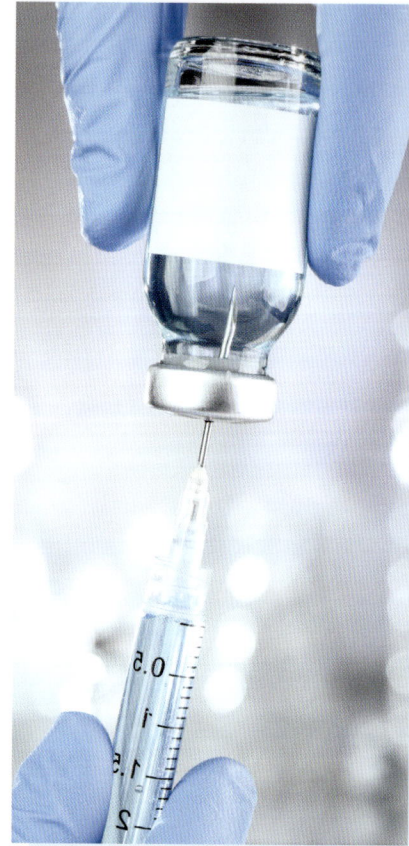

© Leigh Prather/Adobe Stock

> *More parents than ever before are saying no to vitamin K shots.*

In 1990 (the year before the CDC pushed for hepatitis B vaccination of all newborns), the U.S. reported 661 cases of hepatitis B in children age 14 and under.[123] By 2006, the CDC- and FDA-administered Vaccine Adverse Event Reporting System (VAERS) had received over 23,000 reports of adverse events related to hepatitis B vaccination in children 0 to 14 years old, including nearly 800 deaths.[124]

From 1991 to 2001 (when hepatitis B shots contained the mercury-based preservative thimerosal), vaccination in early infancy resulted in up to one million U.S. children being diagnosed with learning disabilities, representing lifetime costs in excess of $1 trillion.[125] Studies link other hepatitis B vaccine ingredients (including aluminum adjuvants and yeast) as well as the shots' use of genetic engineering technology to a variety of adverse outcomes.[126,127,128]

In 2018, author and autism parent JB Handley described a biological study in mice conducted by Chinese researchers. Assessing the effects of neonatal hepatitis B vaccination on brain development, the research team found that the aluminum-containing vaccine led to a spike in a biomarker for autism and produced neurological impacts that often took time to show up.[129] The study was one of three conducted by the Chinese group and, according to Handley, the three studies together represent "clear, unequivocal, replicable scientific evidence that the first vaccine given to most American newborns causes brain damage."[130]

> " By 2006, the CDC- and FDA-administered Vaccine Adverse Event Reporting System (VAERS) had received over 23,000 reports of adverse events related to hepatitis B vaccination in children 0 to 14 years old, including nearly 800 deaths. "

© Wavebreak Media Micro/Adobe Stock

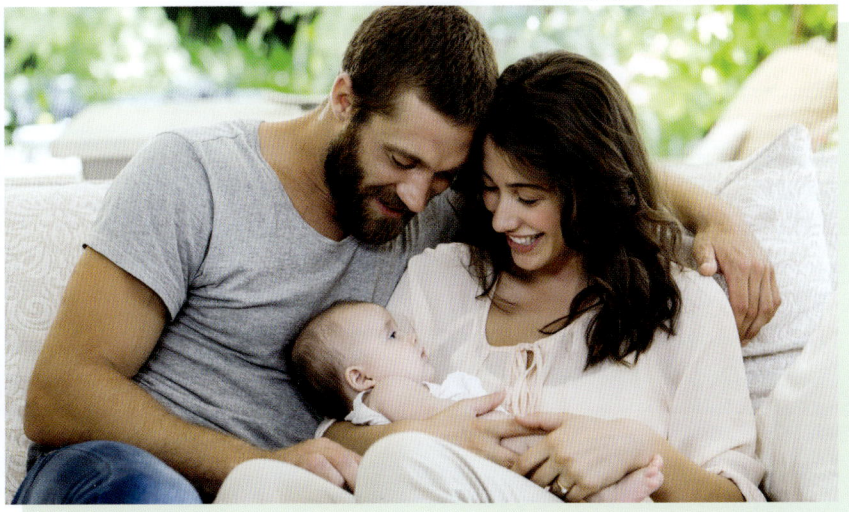

The package inserts for hepatitis B vaccines also include other information that parents may not know about. For example, the package insert for the Engerix-B vaccine manufactured by GlaxoSmithKline (GSK) states in Section 5.3:

> "Hepatitis B vaccine should be deferred for infants with a birth weight <2,000 g if the mother is documented to be HBsAg [hepatitis B surface antigen] negative at the time of the infant's birth. Vaccination can commence at chronological age 1 month or hospital discharge. ... The birth dose in infants born weighing <2,000 g should not be counted as the first dose in the vaccine series and it should be followed with a full 3-dose standard regiment (total of 4 doses)." [131]

Stated another way, this means that the smallest and most vulnerable infants (those born weighing less than 2,000 grams or 4.4 pounds), who will most likely already be struggling with other medical issues, will receive an extra dose of the vaccine compared to their peers who weigh over 4.4 lbs!

The package insert for the Recombivax vaccine made by Merck states (Section 2.1) that persons age 0 through 19 should receive a "series of 3 doses (0.5 mL each) given on a 0-, 1-, and 6-month schedule." [132] In other words, clinicians give the hepatitis B vaccine according to age rather than weight, such that a 4.5-pound neonate will receive the same dosage as a 10-pound neonate. Similarly, an 11-year-old child will receive the same dosage as a 15-year-old child, despite the weight difference.

Both the Engerix-B (Section 5.4) and Recombivax inserts (Section 5.2) state that "Apnea [cessation of breathing] following intramuscular vaccination has been observed in some infants born prematurely."

For breastfeeding mothers who receive hepatitis B shots, both companies (Section 8.2) also acknowledge that there are no data pertaining to the presence of vaccine in human breast milk and no studies assessing possible effects on the breastfeeding baby or on milk production.

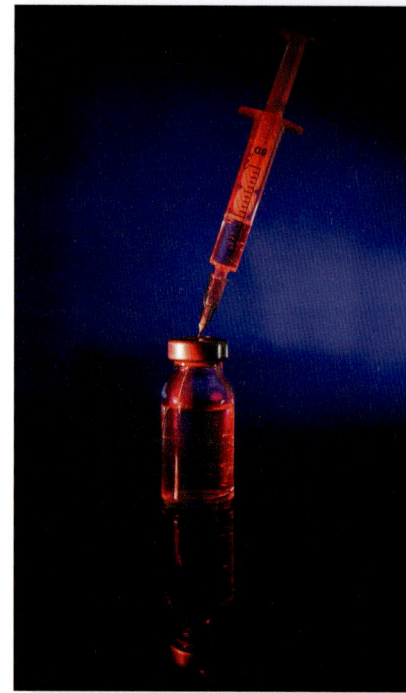

© ADDICTIVE STOCK CORE/Adobe Stock

Clinicians give the hepatitis B vaccine according to age rather than weight, such that a 4.5-pound neonate will receive the same dosage as a 10-pound neonate.

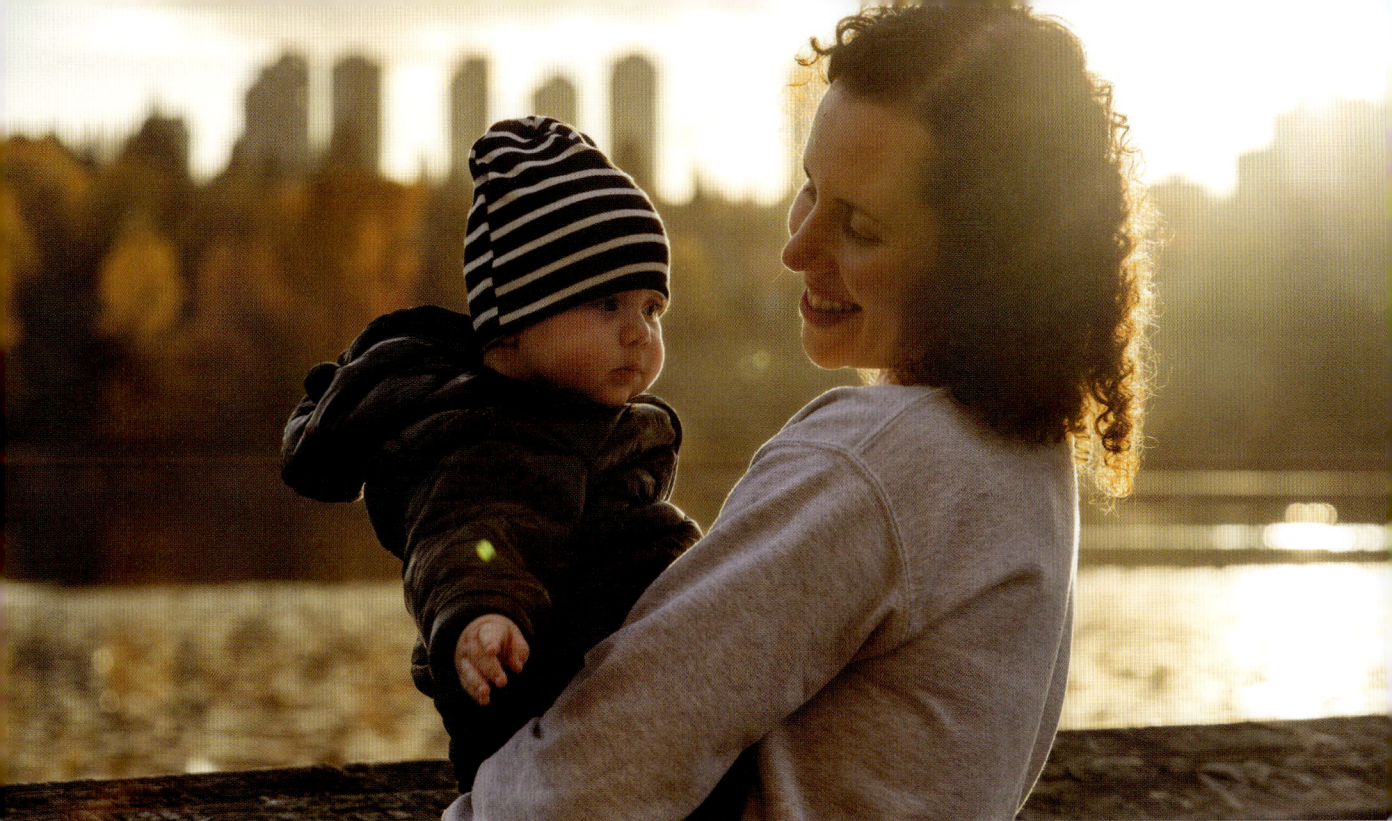

Chapter Four: The First Year

"Every nerve ending under his newly exposed skin craves the expected embrace; all his being, the character of all he is, leads to his being held in arms." — **Jean Liedloff,** *The Continuum Concept* **(1986)**

Within a few hours of birth, a baby can already recognize parents' voices. Within a few days, a baby knows the mother's smell and can identify her face. Babies have the innate will to reach toward the world, represented by reaching for their mother. This is the impulse to be alive, learn, and become.[133]

During the first month, a baby will grow daily and meet developmental milestones rapidly. Just as we experience the rhythm of seasons and sunrise to sunset, newborns experience the rhythm of slow and steady growth and development. Parents' support for babies as they adapt to this new rhythm will allow for optimal health and growth. Ideally, mothers will dedicate the first month to the rhythm of mother and infant adapting and responding to one another during feeding and holding. At the same time, maternal self-care is crucial in keeping a mother healthy and present for her baby and other loved ones.

> 66
>
> *Babies have the innate will to reach toward the world, represented by reaching for their mother.*
>
> 99

In this chapter, we will:

- Describe factors that positively influence a baby's health, including touch, breastfeeding, and bedsharing
- Review newborn reflexes and breathing patterns
- Acknowledge changes that occur in the mother, including some women's experience of postpartum depression
- Discuss the likely link between sudden infant death syndrome (SIDS) and vaccination

Therapeutic Touch

A baby spends approximately 280 days in the womb. The moment of birth is the moment babies are on their own for the first time. A baby looks for constant contact with his or her mother to cope with the separation from the womb. The connection between mother and baby is essential to the development of the child's mind, body, and spirit. Mothers need to pay attention to what their baby is telling them and respond in ways that are right for both.

After birth, infants' primary needs center around warmth, touch, comfort, and nourishment. Many researchers recognize skin-to-skin contact as the glue in the bonding process.[134] Studies show that babies who have the opportunity to bond in this way after birth are physically healthier, more secure, and more active than babies who do not.

In addition to maternal benefits, skin-to-skin bonding also has benefits for fathers or other caregivers. Safe baby wraps and slings can make bonding easier and allow for mobility while carrying a baby. Massaging a baby's skin will also help fulfill their need for contact and bring trust and cooperation into the relationship.

> *A baby looks for constant contact with his or her mother to cope with the separation from the womb.*

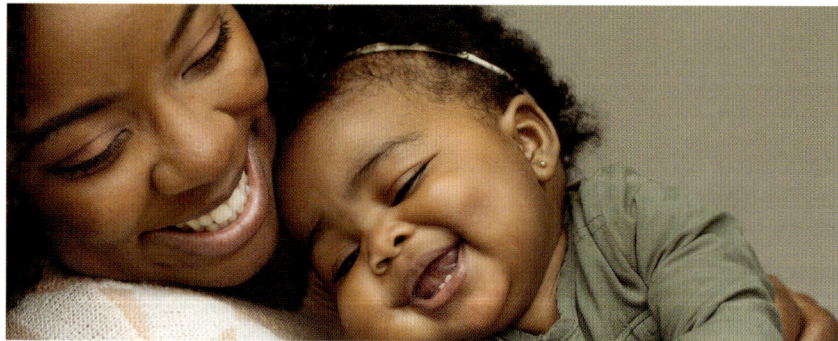

© digitalskillet1/Adobe Stock

The Infant Gut Microbiome and the Benefits of Breastfeeding

The intestines house an ecosystem of about 100 trillion living microorganisms, including bacteria, viruses, and fungi that play important roles such as breaking down food, synthesizing vitamins, and defending against pathogens. This ecosystem is known as the intestinal microbiome.[135]

The infant gut microbiome is not as diverse as an adult's. In the first year of life, the newborn intestinal tract undergoes rapid microbial colonization, with "dramatic changes in the composition of the intestinal microbiome" that vary from infant to infant.[136] Maternal factors—such as stress, medications, or obesity—as well as neonatal factors such as surgical birth, exposure to antibiotics (either in utero or postnatally), and feeding patterns can significantly influence infant microbiome development and gut health.[137] For example, the gut flora of infants born vaginally will be similar to the mother's vaginal flora, whereas C-section delivery will alter the microbial balance. Other environmental insults during the immediate postpartum period, such as malnutrition or illness, can also disrupt optimal microbial colonization. This can contribute to "lifelong and intergenerational deficits in growth and development."[138]

The newborn diet, and breastfeeding in particular, plays an important role in establishing a healthy microbiome in babies, which in turn has long-term implications for overall health.[139] The CDC, AAP, and WHO all recommend exclusive breastfeeding for approximately six months or even longer.[140] When the mother is eating well herself, breast milk is a natural source of a wide range of nutrients unique to a mother and her baby, including beneficial prebiotic human milk oligosaccharides that support the developing infant gut microbiota.[141] A 2020 study confirmed the benefits of bacteria shared through breast milk, finding that feeding directly from the breast is the best way to support the transfer of beneficial organisms.[142] A non-direct mode of breast milk delivery such as breast pumping can affect the bacterial composition of breast milk.[143]

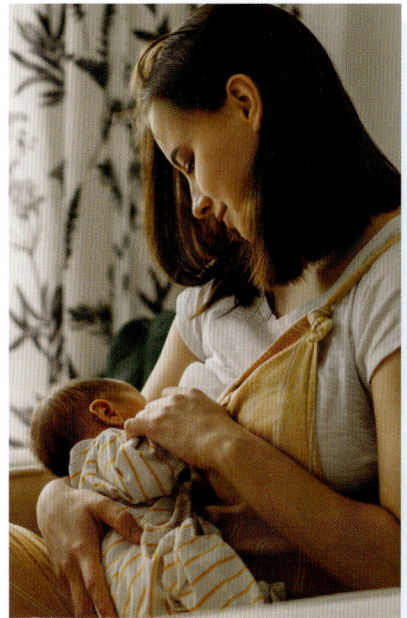

© Anastiasiya Styanailo/Adobe Stock

> *The newborn diet, and breastfeeding in particular, plays an important role in establishing a healthy microbiome in babies, which in turn has long-term implications for overall health.*

If the mother's diet is filled with "sugar, white flour, additives and commercial fats and oils, which do not nourish and build," her breast milk will not provide proper nourishment.[144] However, assuming a well-nourished mother, breastfeeding offers multiple benefits for growing infants:[145]

- Developing a healthy emotional bond with the mother
- Taking in the sum of nutrients that an infant needs
- Acquiring immunity from diseases and allergies

Breast milk helps build and support a baby's immune system by providing protection against common allergies and respiratory and gastrointestinal infections.[146] Breastfeeding and an appropriately diverse gut microbiome also decrease the risk of chronic health conditions such as asthma and allergies,[147] type 1 and type 2 diabetes,[148] inflammatory bowel disease,[149] celiac disease,[150] autoimmune disorders,[151] and some childhood cancers.[152]

In an interesting 2021 study published in the *Journal of Translational Science*,[153] Children's Health Defense chief scientist Brian S. Hooker and coauthor Neil Z. Miller confirmed the protective effects of breastfeeding, particularly in unvaccinated children. They examined the prevalence of six "adverse health conditions" (allergies, autism, asthma, chronic ear infections, gastrointestinal disorders, and attention-deficit disorder/attention-deficit/hyperactivity disorder [ADD/ADHD]) in partially and fully vaccinated versus unvaccinated children and also assessed the influence of breastfeeding and type of birth (vaginal versus C-section). For all six conditions, the "unvaccinated and breastfed" and "unvaccinated and vaginal delivery" groups had the lowest odds of having a diagnosed condition—whereas children who were "vaccinated and not breastfed" or "vaccinated and delivered via C-section" had a significantly higher odds of a diagnosed

> *Breast milk helps build and support a baby's immune system by providing protection against common allergies and respiratory and gastrointestinal infections.*

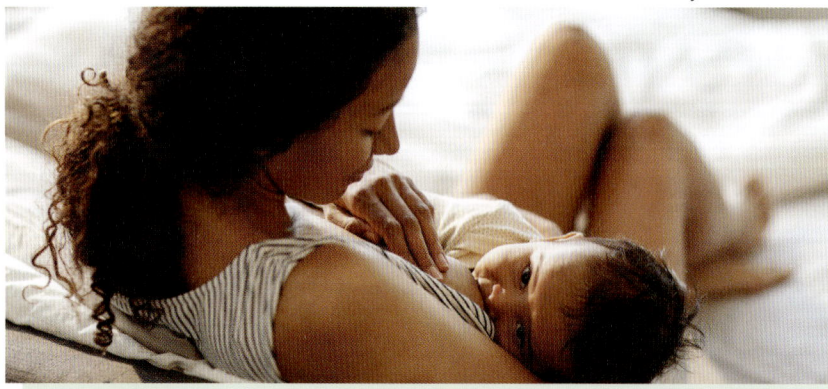

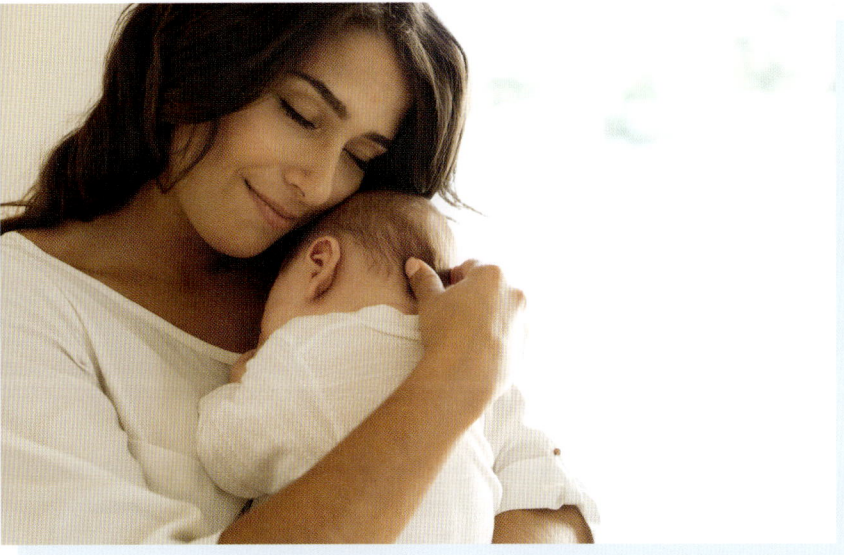

> *A pregnant woman's microbiome "is associated with both the health of the mother as well as the developing fetus."*

condition. The two authors also noted that "vaccination appears to decrease the beneficial effects of breastfeeding, as indicated by the higher proportions of diagnoses in the 'vaccinated and breastfed' group of children as compared to the 'unvaccinated and breastfed' group."

In a separate analysis that just looked at the influence of breastfeeding, they found that breastfed children "were less likely to be diagnosed with allergies, asthma and ear infections," while a separate analysis focusing on type of birth found that diagnosed gastrointestinal disorders were "more common in children delivered via C-section."

Antibiotics and the Microbiome

It is by now common knowledge that even a single course of antibiotics can wreak havoc on the gut flora,[154] creating an environment in which pathogenic bacteria and fungi proliferate, no longer held in check by the beneficial flora wiped out by the drugs.[155] It is also well known that a pregnant woman's microbiome "is associated with both the health of the mother as well as the developing fetus."[156] Studies have linked prenatal antibiotics to health problems in offspring that include newborn thrush and yeast infections,[157] allergic conditions,[158] childhood obesity,[159] and neurological conditions like ADHD and epilepsy,[160] among others.

47

Despite the potential risks for infants, at least 20% to 25% of women are given antibiotics during pregnancy.[161] This includes a blanket antibiotics recommendation for women who test "positive" for group B strep (GBS) (normal bacteria found in up to 30% of women that pose a "very small" risk of passing to and making the infant sick[162]), despite mounting evidence that this intervention is both ineffective and harmful.[163] Fortunately, there are numerous natural alternatives that can help pregnant women prevent a positive GBS test altogether or eliminate GBS bacteria after a positive test as well as offering options for labor; these include probiotics, vitamin C supplementation, vaginal rinses with apple cider vinegar, garlic vaginal suppositories, herbal tinctures, and more.[164]

Doctors also routinely administer antibiotics to women who undergo C-sections.[165] Unfortunately, according to researchers at the University of California, Davis (UC-Davis), antibiotic overuse and the rise in cesarean births have contributed to the near-eradication in American infants of *B. infantis*, "a strain of bacteria ... thought to have been the dominant bacterium in the infant gut for all of human history."[166] When *B. infantis* predominates in the infant gut, the researchers note, "it crowds all the other guys out," including pathogenic bacteria, but when it is missing, children are more likely to develop allergies and other chronic ailments.

> *Despite the potential risks for infants, at least 20% to 25% of women are given antibiotics during pregnancy.*

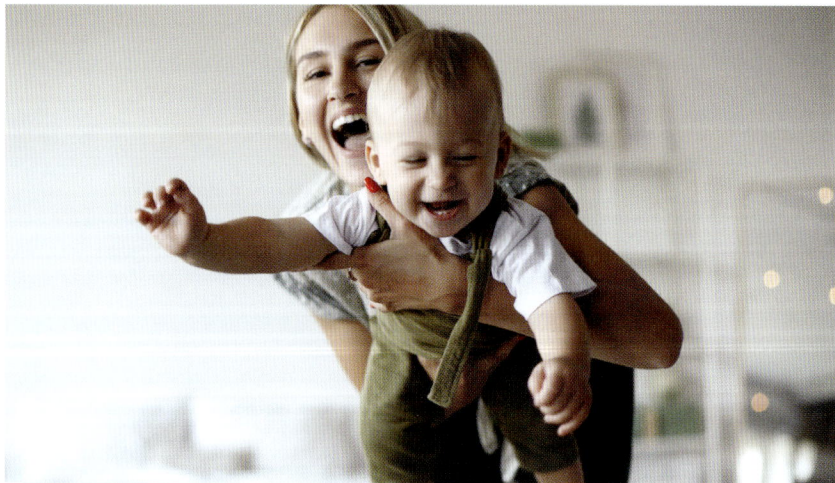

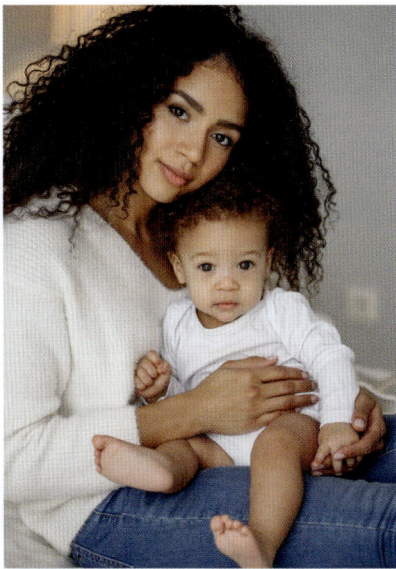
© Miramiska/Adobe Stock

Breastfeeding Challenges and Alternatives

Breastfeeding is not a one-size-fits-all approach. For some mothers, breastfeeding can be intimidating and overwhelming as they attempt to navigate other new challenges at the same time. In the fast-paced modern world, women may also face socio-economic barriers that make breastfeeding difficult.[169] Some women may endure extreme pressure to juggle academic, career, and maternal aspirations. Mothers may also encounter breastfeeding difficulties, such as challenges in getting their infant to latch properly. Some mothers have low milk production or a medical condition that limits their ability to breastfeed. Even so, primary lactation failure and medical contraindications are relatively rare.

Many community resources are available to support breastfeeding mothers, including lactation consultants and postpartum doulas.[170,171] It can be helpful to explore or line up support options *before* the birth, so that assistance will be at hand in case of subsequent need.

Even formula manufacturers recognize that *B. infantis* has a "symbiotic relationship" with the human host "that protects the preterm or term neonate and nourishes a healthy gut microbiota prior to weaning."[167] However, formula feeding has contributed to the disappearance of *B. infantis*, because the bacteria's nourishment relies on carbohydrates unique to breast milk. The UC Davis research group and a probiotics manufacturer reported in 2022 in *Pediatric Research* that *B. infantis* probiotic supplementation within a month of birth, "in combination with breast milk, resulted in stable colonization that persisted until at least 1 year postnatal."[168]

> *Mothers may also encounter breastfeeding difficulties, such as challenges in getting their infant to latch properly.*

Feeding should be comfortable for the mother. Sometimes, when milk becomes trapped in the breast, a condition called mastitis can develop—causing inflammation, pain, redness, tenderness, fever, flu-like symptoms, and/or swelling of one or both breasts.[172] Bacteria from the skin's surface and the baby's mouth can enter the milk ducts through cracks in the skin of a nipple or through a milk duct opening. Stagnant milk in a breast that isn't emptied can provide a breeding ground for the bacteria.[173] Fortunately, there are ways to prevent inflammation and decrease the risk of mastitis and infection.

For women who, for various reasons, cannot directly breastfeed but want to nourish their baby with breast milk, alternatives include exclusive breast pumping and donor milk.[174,175] (Mothers should know that donated human milk from milk banks is pasteurized.) Two other alternatives in addition to human milk are homemade formula and commercial formula. The Weston A. Price Foundation recipes for homemade formula,[176] carefully developed by nutrition pioneer and lipids expert Dr. Mary Enig,[177] have helped babies thrive for over two decades.[178]

According to Drugwatch.com, a website that provides information on high-risk pharmaceutical products and legal actions, there may be concerns with formulas produced in the United States.[179] The 2022 recall of formula manufactured by Abbott underscored the basis for some of these consumer worries.[180] As a result, some American parents choose to purchase European baby formula to avoid potential harms.[181] However, in both Europe and the U.S., manufacturers are now turning to synthetic biology and biotech to make formula ingredients; for example, many formulas now feature a highly synthetic substance called 2'-FL produced using genetically modified strains of *Escherichia coli*.[182]

> *Two other alternatives in addition to human milk are homemade formula and commercial formula.*

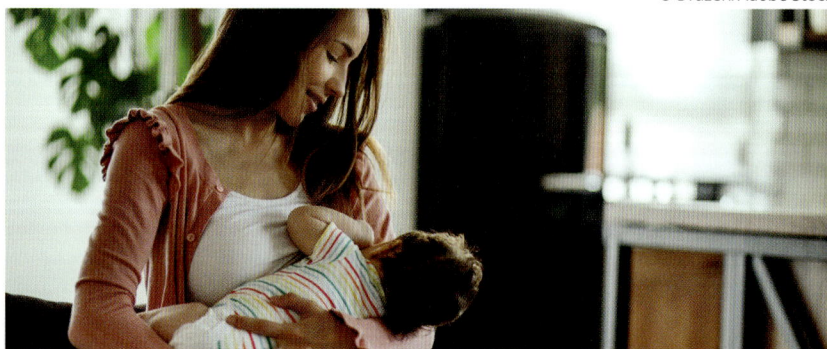

If using commercial formula, an organic, additive-free, soy-free formula is preferable.[183] Compounds called phytoestrogens in soy formula can accelerate puberty and cause reproductive and thyroid disorders later in life, and researchers have also linked soy formula to seizures and autism.[184,185] Other problems with soy formula include the manufacturing process—which introduces neurotoxic, carcinogenic, and excitotoxic byproducts—and a high aluminum content.[186,187]

Determining Whether Baby Is Getting Enough Milk

It is nearly impossible to measure the milk from breastfeeding. So, how will a breastfeeding mother know if her baby is getting enough?

Although every baby is different, in the first month, a baby generally should be nursing 8 to 12 times per day (every 2 to 3 hours) in a 24-hour period, with feedings lasting anywhere from 5 to 40 minutes. A breastfeeding baby should be taking deep rhythmic sucks and swallowing hard throughout the feeding. Babies will come off the breast by themselves when satisfied. Feeding replenishes a woman's milk supply; the more a baby breastfeeds, the more milk the mother produces. Infants will eat when they are hungry. Parents can observe infants' desire for food as the first step in determining if they are taking in enough.

> " Although every baby is different, in the first month, a baby generally should be nursing 8 to 12 times per day. "

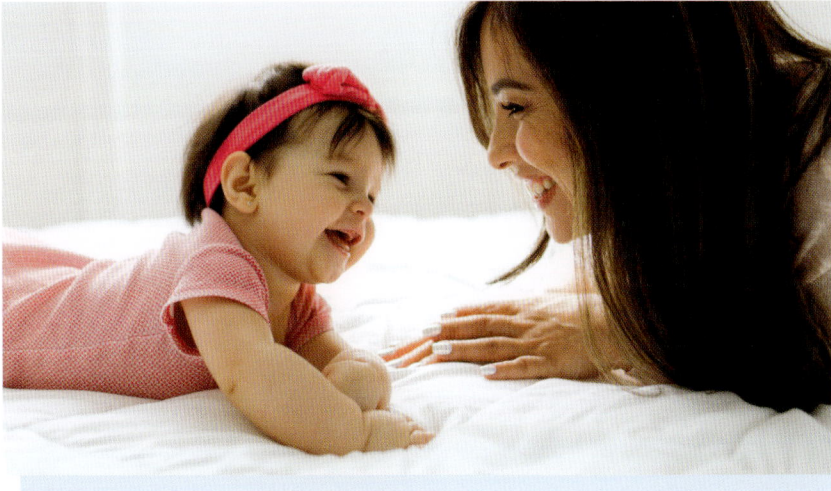

© AntonioDiaz/Adobe Stock

For a newborn who is bottle-feeding, about 1.5 to 3 ounces (45–90 milliliters) are appropriate every two to three hours. This amount increases as a baby grows and is able to take more at each feeding. At about two months, a baby may take 4 to 5 ounces (120–150 milliliters) at each feeding, and the feedings may stretch out to every three to four hours.

A well-fed baby produces about six wet diapers a day and about two stools. A baby should be content and happy after each feeding. Babies should be awake, alert, and meeting developmental mile-stones while also growing out of their clothes. As a mother and baby bond, the mother will begin to feel more comfortable in knowing when her baby is experiencing satiety — the feeling of fullness after eating. Trusting maternal intuition is key. If a mother senses that her baby is continuously irritable after feedings, has decreased wet diapers, or is unable to gain weight, she should consider seeking trusted medical advice.

> " *A well-fed baby produces about six wet diapers a day and about two stools.* "

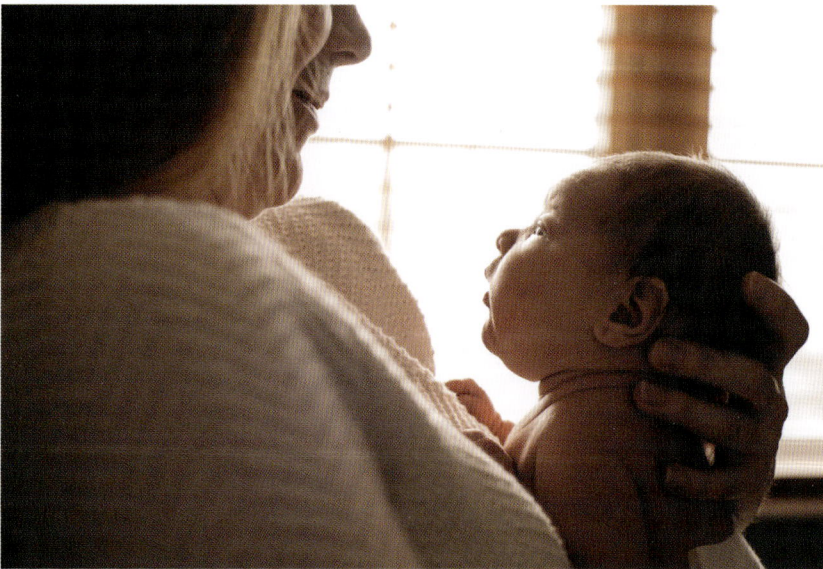

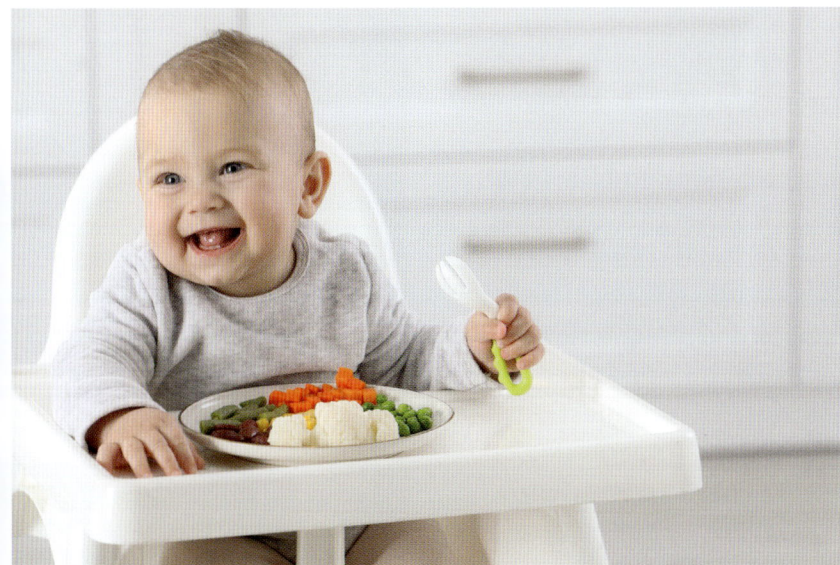
© New Africa/Adobe Stock

> It has become common for infants to have intermittent spit-ups following both breastfeeding and bottle feeding.

Gastroesophageal Reflux

"My infant will spit up a teaspoon full of breast milk about three times daily after feeding, is this normal?"

Due to a general decline in adults' and children's digestive health in Western nations,[188] it has become common for infants to have intermittent spit-ups following both breastfeeding and bottle feeding. One estimate suggests that 65% of infants regurgitate stomach contents at least once daily between the ages of three and six months, although four out of five babies outgrow the behavior by six months.[189] This phenomenon is known as physiologic gastroesophageal reflux (GER) or "acid reflux." GER is particularly common in babies born prematurely.[190]

Spitting up is often upsetting to parents and can also be inconvenient, requiring frequent changes of clothes. Although doctors generally tell parents that as long as the baby is content and growing well, reflux is not a cause for concern, acid reflux is invariably a sign of poor digestion,[191] is uncomfortable for babies, and can contribute to colic.[192]

Physiologically, between the esophagus and the stomach is a portal called the lower esophageal sphincter (LES). Normally, when someone swallows, the food travels down the esophagus, and the sphincter relaxes, permitting the food to enter the stomach where a pool of acid awaits to continue digesting it. The sphincter then closes tightly. In most newborns, the LES is relatively lax and not fully mature, which can allow for stomach contents to easily flow back up. As "obligate nasal breathers," babies must learn to suck and swallow while breathing through the nose. A baby also needs to gain muscle tone to be able to sit up for easier digestion. Eventually, the LES will open only when the baby swallows and will remain tightly closed at other times, keeping stomach contents where they belong.

Breastfeeding mothers can improve their infant's digestion by strengthening their own gut health and eating a nutrient-dense diet rich in probiotic foods. Other steps that parents can take to prevent or manage GER include not feeding babies in a supine (lying down) position, keeping babies upright for one hour after feeding (for example, in a sling or wrap), and feeding babies more often but with less volume at each feeding.

Reflux medications are of "questionable efficacy and safety."[193] Parents should avoid giving their infants proton pump inhibitors (PPIs) or H2 blockers that reduce stomach acid; these drugs come with significant risks, including dysregulation of the gut flora, food allergies, gastrointestinal infections, and adverse impacts on bone health.[194] Moreover, there is no evidence that stomach acid plays any role in patterns of unsettledness, irritability, or reflux in infancy or that acid suppression does anything to improve these distressing behaviors. On the contrary, stomach acid (also called gastric acid) prevents unwanted bacterial growth in the stomach and upper intestine, and helps babies digest the nutrients in their food or milk appropriately.

That said, it is important to distinguish between physiologic GER in infants and gastroesophageal reflux disease (GERD). If an infant is failing to gain weight, is consistently irritable after feeding, refuses food, has blood in their stool, has a chronic cough or difficulty breathing, or has progressive projectile vomiting after every feeding despite interventions to mitigate reflux, it is probably time to consult a trusted medical professional.

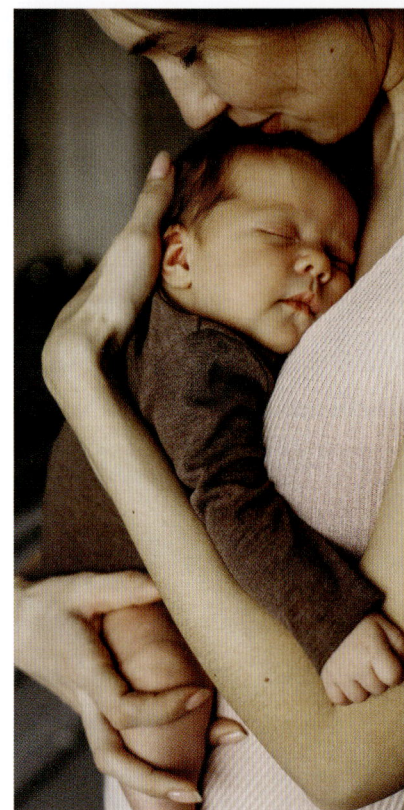

© annaperevozkina/Adobe Stock

A baby also needs to gain muscle tone to be able to sit up for easier digestion.

Newborn Reflexes

Babies arrive well-equipped with reflexes that help support them through the first couple of months of life and provide the foundation for more complex reflex schemes later in life. According to Svetlana Masgutova, creator of the Masgutova Neurosensorimotor Reflex Integration (MNRI) Method, infant reflexes play a major role "in maturation, development, and normal life function" and do not so much disappear as "integrate."[195] The newborn reflexes are a common assessment tool that healthcare providers use to evaluate infants.[196]

Blinking Reflex

Babies are sensitive to bright lights. When babies encounter a flash of light or a puff of air near the eyes, their eyes will close. This blinking reflex is permanent and will stick with the child throughout their life.

Babinski Reflex

An adult can elicit the Babinski reflex by gently stroking the sole of a baby's foot with a finger or a soft object. The baby's toes will fan out, with the foot perhaps twisting inward. This reflex typically disappears after nine months to one year.

> *When babies encounter a flash of light or a puff of air near the eyes, their eyes will close.*

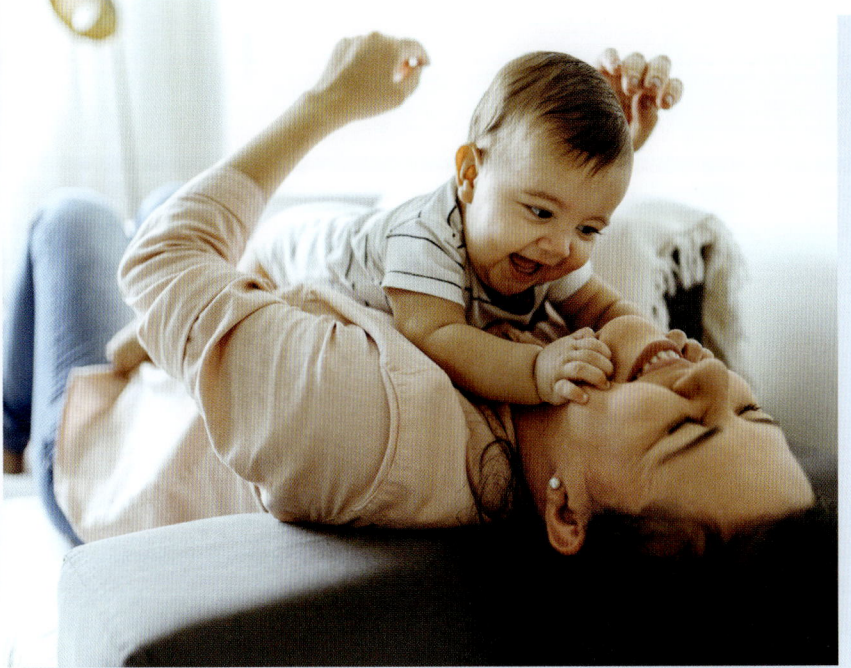

© kleberpicui/Adobe Stock

Grasping Reflex

An infant may grab tightly onto the mother's finger—this is the grasping reflex. An adult can elicit the reflex by touching the palm of the right or left hand. This reflex begins to weaken after three months and then disappears after one year of age.

Moro Reflex

Hearing a loud noise or experiencing the sensation of falling (such as when being put down) stimulates the Moro reflex, also known as the startle reflex. Babies will arch their back and throw their head back, flinging out arms and legs, and then rapidly curl them to the center of the body. This reflex should disappear after three to six months of age.

Rooting Reflex

When infants are hungry, they will turn their head to the side and open their mouth as an indication that it's time to feed. Caregivers can elicit this rooting reflex by touching the cheek or side of the mouth. If an infant is often sleepy, stroking the side of the cheek or mouth will usually help them to be ready to eat. It is not uncommon for this reflex to disappear at around three to four months of age.

Sucking Reflex

Placing a nipple or pacifier near a baby's mouth elicits the sucking reflex. This is an essential reflex as it allows a baby to consume nourishment.

> *When infants are hungry, they will turn their head to the side and open their mouth as an indication that it's time to feed.*

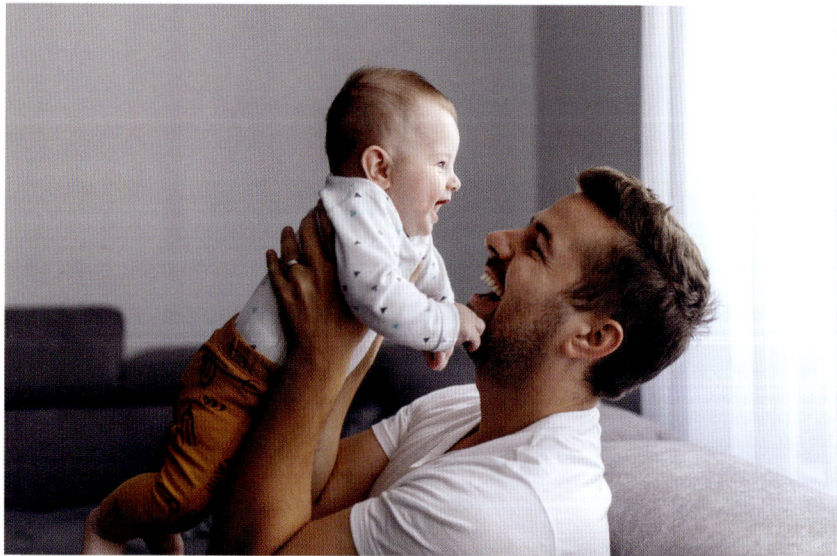

© Dusan Petkovic/Adobe Stock

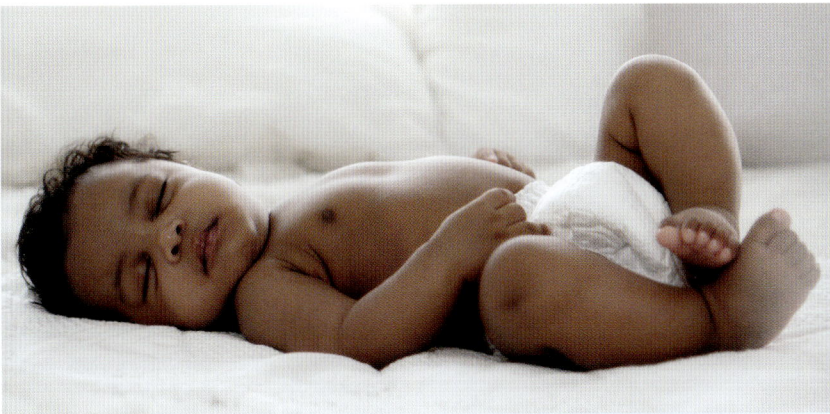

© Mongkolchon/Adobe Stock

Stepping Reflex

Another reflex that disappears after three to four months is the stepping reflex. If an adult holds an infant gently above a flat surface and slowly lowers them onto their feet, the infant should move their feet as if they are trying to walk or "step."

Tonic Neck Reflex

It is possible to elicit the tonic neck reflex, also known as the "fencing" position, when a baby is lying on his or her back. If the baby's head is turned to one side, the arm on that side stretches out and the opposite arm bends up at the elbow. This reflex typically disappears around six to seven months of age.

Infant Breathing

From the moment a baby comes out of the womb, parents wait eagerly to hear that first cry. However, many new parents become hyper-vigilant out of fear that their baby, when sleeping, will stop breathing. This parental concern is so common that companies have made breathing monitors; sometimes, however, these monitors can be counterproductive, eliciting even more of a fear and anxiety response.

> "
> *From the moment a baby comes out of the womb, parents wait eagerly to hear that first cry.*
> "

To allay parental concerns, it can be helpful to understand infants' unique physiological breathing patterns and to know that a baby's breathing pattern is different from an adult's.[197] An adult's breathing rate is normally about 12 to 20 breaths per minute, but a newborn will take inhalations and exhalations about 30 to 60 times per minute, slowing to 30 to 40 breaths per minute when sleeping. As a baby grows, breathing rates slowly decrease. By about six months of age, a baby may breathe about 25 to 40 times per minute.

The fact that infants are obligate nose breathers sometimes is concerning for new parents. However, even beyond infancy, breathing through the nose continues to be important for good health. Nasal breathing "forces air to get heated, pressurized, filtered, and conditioned, allowing the lungs to extract oxygen much more efficiently," while oral (mouth) breathing jettisons those benefits.[198] Asthma researchers have suggested that mouth breathing reduces lung function and may, in fact, contribute to the development of asthma,[199] as well as the occurrence of "acute asthma exacerbations."[200] Studies also point to "more brain activa-

tion and connection during nasal breathing than during oral breathing," indicating that nose breathing is important for cognitive function.[201]

Some signs of respiratory distress may indicate the necessity of medical evaluation:[202]

- Increased breathing rate
- Nasal flaring (an indication that the child is working harder to breathe)
- Noisy breathing such as wheezing, grunting, or high-pitched whistling
- Open mouth
- Blue-tinged skin (especially lips, fingernails, gums, and under eyes)
- Skin pulling in around bones in chest
- Increased coughing
- Difficulty sleeping

In addition, some infants experience irregular breathing patterns called "periodic breathing," which can manifest as faster breathing, unusual sounds, or long pauses between breaths—for three or more seconds at a time. Several such pauses may occur close together, followed by a series of rapid, shallow breaths. This irregular breathing pattern is common in premature babies in the first few weeks of life and can represent a red flag for reduced oxygenation of the brain.[203]

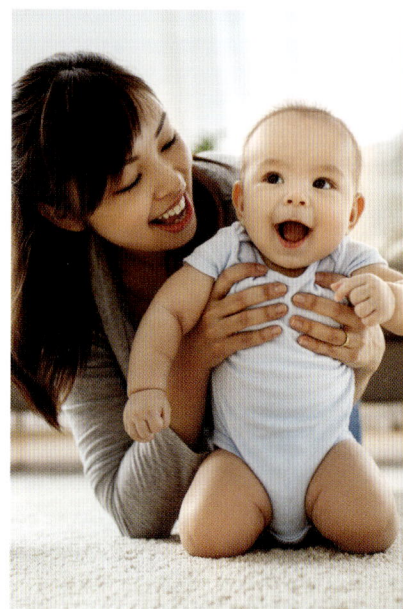

© Syda Productions/Adobe Stock

> Asthma researchers have suggested that mouth breathing reduces lung function and may, in fact, contribute to the development of asthma.

Although conventional medicine has sought to normalize periodic breathing in full-term infants, claiming it is harmless, researchers from the late 1970s on have disagreed. In 1979, researchers documented the presence of periodic breathing "in excessive amounts during sleep in infants with near-miss sudden infant death syndrome" (SIDS), compared to infants in a control group, with a statistically significant difference between the two groups.[204] Beginning in the mid-1980s (1986–1993), Australia-based scientist Viera Scheibner highlighted the "stressed breathing" caused by vaccination as a key culprit for SIDS (which she renamed as "Sudden Immunisation Death Syndrome").[205] Using breathing monitors, she recorded the effect of vaccination "on babies' breathing hour by hour and … demonstrated the existence of …

critical days on which there are flare-ups of stressed breathing caused by [the administered vaccinations]," with "an inordinate increase in episodes where breathing nearly ceased or stopped completely" for several weeks following vaccination.[206] In 1997, researchers reiterated that "periodic breathing in the term infant is not a benign event," arguing that it represents a risk factor for SIDS.[207]

> In 1997, researchers reiterated that "periodic breathing in the term infant is not a benign event," arguing that it represents a risk factor for SIDS.

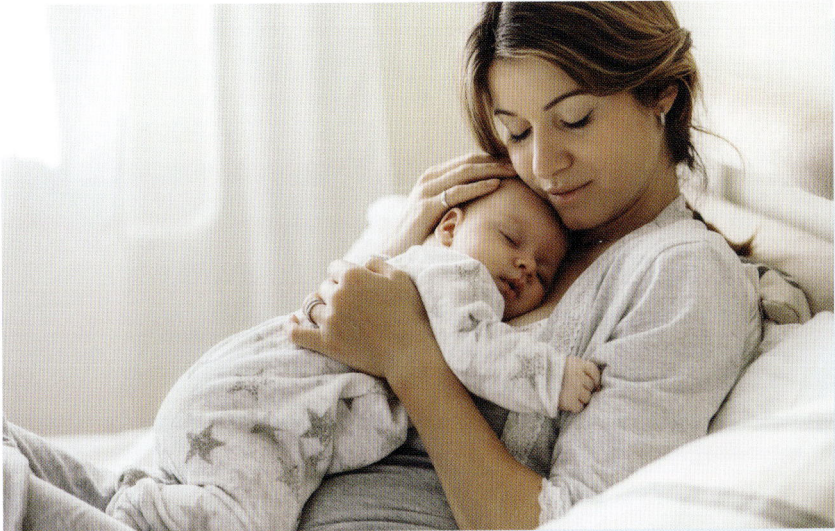

Sleeping: When and Where

"People often ask me how a sailor gets any sleep when ocean racing solo. While sleeping, the lone sailor puts the boat on autopilot. Because the sailor is so in tune with his boat, if the wind shifts so that something is not quite right with the boat, the sailor will wake up."
— **Dr. Jim Sears**

New mothers often observe that their baby seems not to recognize the difference between day and night, and simply alternates between periods of sleeping and eating. It is normal for newborns to sleep 15 to 18 hours in every 24-hour cycle; in fact, according to sleep expert Elizabeth Pantley, "newborns do best with short awake spans interspersed with plenty of naps."[208] Describing babies' sleep systems as "immature," Pantley advises parents not to harbor unreasonable expectations:

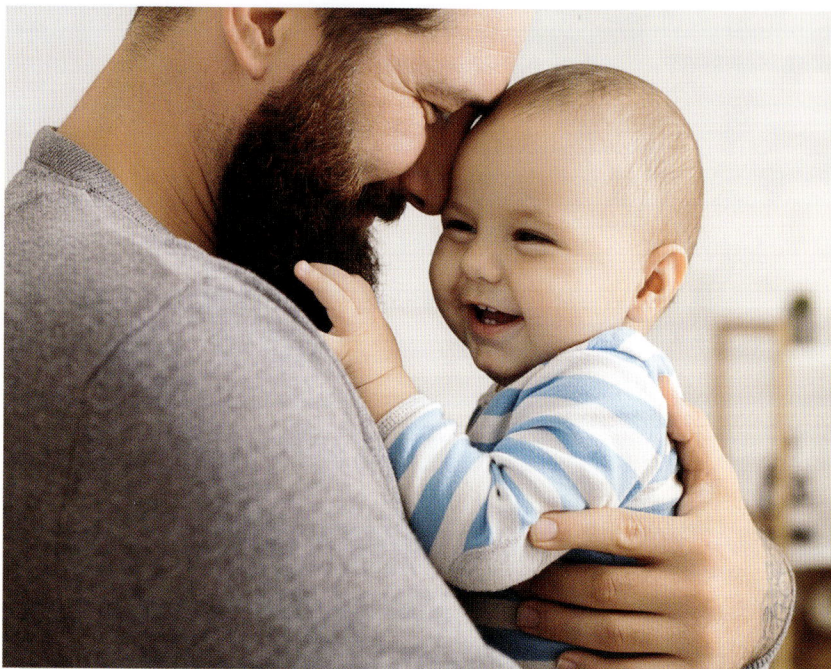

© Prostock-studio/Adobe Stock

"[I]t is perfectly natural, absolutely normal, and totally expected for your baby to wake up in the night and need nourishment or your help to fall back to sleep. Sleeping all through the night, every night, without needing a parent's assistance, is like learning to walk or talk or drink from a cup—all kids get there, but they do so at their own speed, a little bit at a time, and in their own unique way."

> *It is normal for newborns to sleep 15 to 18 hours in every 24-hour cycle.*

Parents with less rigid ideas about infant sleep are generally much happier and far less likely to be disappointed when their children cannot perform the way they are "supposed to," such as sleeping through the night. It may be wise to gently acknowledge the new rhythms and surrender to them. As a mother is adjusting to a new rhythm of living, so is the baby.

When it comes to sleeping arrangements, parents should do their own research and make the decision they feel is best for themselves and their child. Many families develop and exhibit fluid notions of where and when their baby "should" sleep, and three out of five (61%) opt for some bedsharing (also called co-sleeping).[209] Most mothers understand that a strong connection with their baby is important and that skin-to-skin contact is vital. In 2015, referring specifically to bedsharing in conjunction with breastfeeding, sleep expert Drs. James McKenna and Lee Gettler coined the term "breastsleeping," documenting through 25 years of research at the Mother-Baby Behavioral Sleep Laboratory that the two practices are "physiologically and behaviorally interdependent" and together support "optimal infant breastfeeding, neonatal attachment and brain growth."[210] Benefits for mothers also include stronger bonding, more sleep, and better management of their milk supply. Some dentists argue that night nursing contributes to early cavities, but research and empirical observation have discredited this theory,[211] instead showing that "complete breastmilk with all its components" is protective and emphasizing the importance of a nutrient-dense diet in both mother and child.[212,213]

Groups like the AAP and CDC frown on bedsharing, blaming the practice for some of the 3,500 "sleep-related" deaths experienced by U.S. babies annually,[214] including deaths classified as SIDS. However, McKenna and colleagues criticize the organizations' blanket warnings as "scientifically inaccurate and misleading," arguing that feeding method and family context are important variables that need to be taken into account.[215] In the absence of hazards such as parental drug or alcohol use, they show that bedsharing "is not a significant risk factor for SIDS, and after three months of age … may well be protective."[216] They also point out that breastsleeping "adds protection by helping infants to avoid the often dangerous, deeper sleep associated with formula feeding and solitary infant sleep."

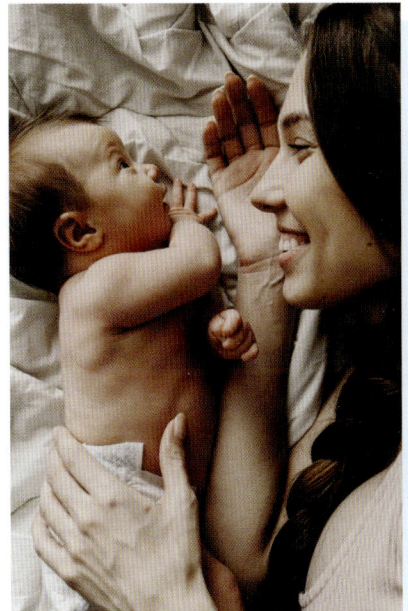

© annaperevozkina/Adobe Stock

> "A strong connection with their baby is important and that skin-to-skin contact is vital."

61

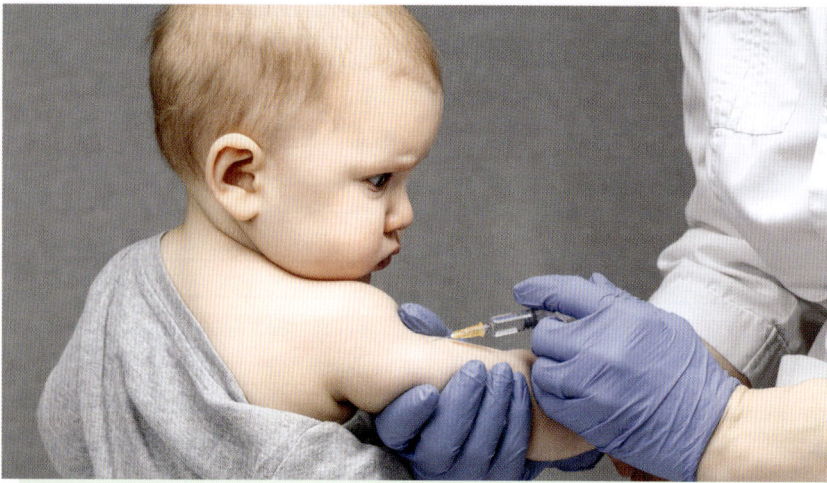

© Dmitry Naumov/Adobe Stock

McKenna's research suggests that a solitary infant sleep environment "represents a neurobiological crisis for the human newborn" and a failure to meet babies' basic needs.[217] Public health officials actually agree with McKenna on this point, acknowledging that sleeping alone in a room is a risk factor for SIDS and endorsing "room sharing" strategies such as placing a bassinet or crib next to the parents' sleeping space.[218] Other "safe sleep" recommendations include keeping the sleep area free of surrounding cushions, stuffed animals, and passive smoke exposure.

Vaccination Risks

As of 2018, children born in the U.S. were 76% more likely to die before their first birthday than infants born in 19 other wealthy nations.[219] Vaccination is a more likely and logical explanation for these sudden baby deaths than bedsharing, but it is an avenue that the CDC and AAP will neither concede nor explore. Clues come from two studies published in 2011 and 2023 by statisticians Neil Miller and Gary Goldman, pointing to a strong correlation between infant mortality rates and number of vaccine doses; countries like the U.S. that administer 21 to 26 vaccine doses during infancy tend to have the highest rates of infant death.[220,221,222]

> " As of 2018, children born in the U.S. were 76% more likely to die before their first birthday than infants born in 19 other wealthy nations. "

SIDS—which, by definition, is the "unexplained, sudden death of a seemingly healthy baby under the age of one"—was and still is one of the top five causes in the U.S.[223] According to the CDC, infant deaths from SIDS and other "unknown causes" represented about 73% of the broader category of sudden unexpected infant deaths (SUID) in 2020, with CDC attributing the remainder (27%) to "accidental suffocation and strangulation in bed."[224]

Historically, it was not until after the launch of various national immunization campaigns that medical certifiers, in the late 1960s, first coined the term "sudden infant death syndrome."[225] In the 1970s, children began receiving 13 vaccines instead of seven and also went from mostly receiving one shot at a time to often getting two at once.[226] The bifurcation between infant mortality in the U.S. versus other rich countries became particularly noticeable in the 1980s,[227] coinciding with a major shift in U.S. infant and childhood vaccination policies, including a strong push to enact and enforce vaccine mandates in schools and, toward the close of the decade, a significant jump in the total number of vaccines required—a trend that continues to this day.

Nowadays, two- and four-month-olds typically receive five or six vaccines at a single "well-baby" appointment, and—with the addition of COVID-19 vaccines to the vaccine schedule starting in the first year of life—may receive as many as eight at a six-month appointment.[228] Between two and four months is exactly the window when nine out of ten SIDS deaths historically have occurred.[229]

In a research paper published in 2021, Miller spelled out the clear temporal relationship: 58% of infant deaths reported to VAERS over three decades (1990–2019) occurred within three days of vaccination, and nearly eight in ten (78%) occurred within a week of vaccination.[230] Moreover, case and pathology reports have identified plausible mechanisms whereby vaccination triggers fatal brain swelling and respiratory distress in infants, including via the vaccines' aluminum adjuvants.[231,232]

> 66
> *SIDS—which, by definition, is the "unexplained, sudden death of a seemingly healthy baby under the age of one"—was and still is one of the top five causes in the U.S.*
> 99

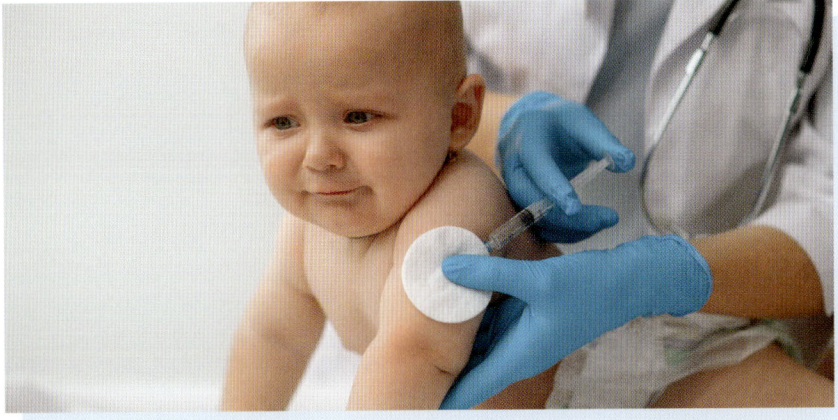

In European studies of SIDS and vaccination, hexavalent ("six-in-one") vaccines have been notable repeat offenders. In 2018, the FDA approved the first six-in-one shot for the U.S. market—a Merck/Sanofi shot called Vaxelis intended as a three-dose series at two, four, and six months—and the U.S. began widespread distribution in 2021. In the Vaxelis arm of the U.S. clinical trials, six infants died within six weeks of receiving Vaxelis, and one infant died in a "control" group given a five-in-one vaccine, with the causes of death reported as SIDS, brain swelling, and abnormal breathing—adverse events identical to those described following hexavalent vaccination in Europe.[233] Vaxelis includes not one but two aluminum adjuvants, including a proprietary "super-powered" adjuvant made by Merck.[234]

Interestingly, after childhood vaccination rates plummeted during the intense lockdowns of 2020, there was a correspondingly precipitous drop in the number of SIDS reports received by VAERS—the lowest yearly number in the adverse event reporting system's history—and a decline in infant mortality generally.[235] Since 2020, there has been a growing trend toward increased parental refusal of some or all childhood vaccines.[236]

SIDS is far from the only vaccine adverse event of concern. In their comparisons of health conditions in vaccinated and unvaccinated children, Hooker and Miller found that vaccination during the first year of life was associated with increased odds of developmental delays, asthma, and ear infections (otitis media) by age three, and increased odds of gastrointestinal disorders by age five—and the more vaccine doses that infants received, the higher the odds.[237] A 2017 study by researcher Anthony R. Mawson and coauthors produced similar findings for children ages 6 to 12, showing that vaccinated children "were significantly more likely to have been diagnosed with otitis media, pneumonia, allergic rhinitis, eczema, and [neurodevelopmental disorders]."[238] As with the Hooker and Miller research, the number of doses made a difference; "the partially vaccinated had increased but intermediate odds of chronic disease, between those of unvaccinated and fully vaccinated children." Related research also suggests that "vaccines are not only associated with adverse health outcomes—they are also associated with more severe and chronic adverse health outcomes."[239]

> *Since 2020, there has been a growing trend toward increased parental refusal of some or all childhood vaccines.*

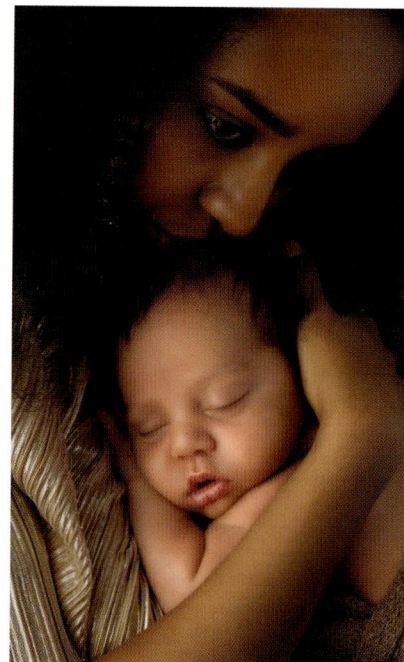

© Anneke/Adobe Stock

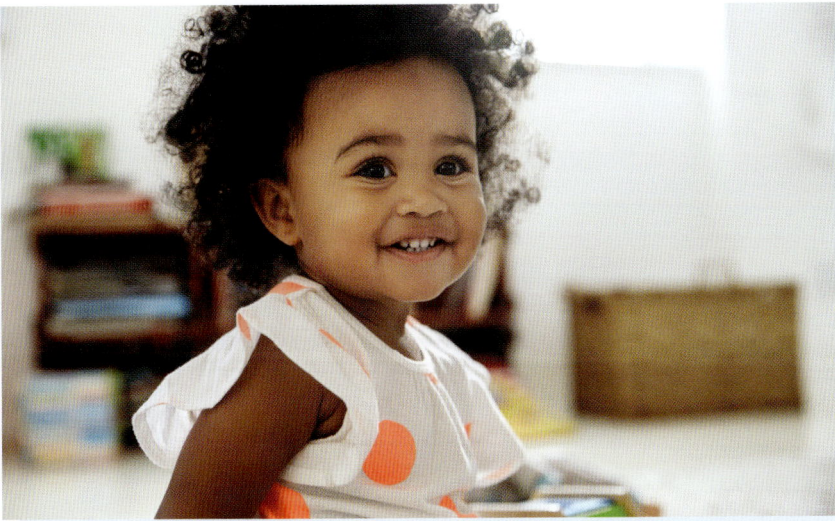

© Monkey Business/Adobe Stock

> *A baby's skin is delicate, and anything placed on an infant's skin will be absorbed into the body.*

Skin: The Largest Organ

Parents may find it confusing to make decisions regarding skin care for their baby. A good guiding principle is that less may be more and simple is often best.

A baby's skin is delicate, and anything placed on an infant's skin will be absorbed into the body. There is no need for fancy or expensive products that claim to be "safe" but often are loaded with toxins and chemicals. Harsh soaps may also contain toxic ingredients. Even baby lotions that claim to be organic, sensitive, or "pure" often contain hidden toxins. According to one "eco" website, baby care products expose the average baby to 27 chemicals a day—and as if that were not bad enough, none of those chemicals have ever "been assessed for safety by industry or government."[240] If the ingredients listed on the bottle are unpronounceable, it may not be safe to use that product.

Diaper rash is one of the most common skin issues parents encounter. Potential causes of diaper rash include irritation from contact with stool and urine, overgrowth of yeast (*Candida albicans*), and conditions such as eczema or seborrhea. Other risk factors for diaper rash include formula allergies, age (being 6–9 months old), diarrhea, antibiotics that cause diarrhea, or transitioning to solid food.[241]

The best and simplest remedies for diaper rash are natural, with the most effective treatment and prevention being simply to keep a baby's bottom clean and dry.[242] This includes changing a baby's diaper frequently (six to eight times per day), avoiding plastic pants that reduce air circulation to the diaper area, and regularly allowing a baby's bottom to be exposed to air and sunlight. Plain water, mild soap, or hypoallergenic wipes are all preferable to diaper wipes that contain alcohol, perfumes, or chemicals, which can sting broken or irritated skin.

Coconut oil is a great skin protector for a baby's bottom after diaper changes, especially for a yeast-related diaper rash; topical application of arrowroot powder or bentonite clay can also help babies stay dry. It is best to avoid commercial baby powders. In 2020, tens of thousands of lawsuits forced Johnson & Johnson (J&J) to stop selling its well-known baby powder due to its inclusion of asbestos—a fact that J&J reportedly knew but hid for decades.[243]

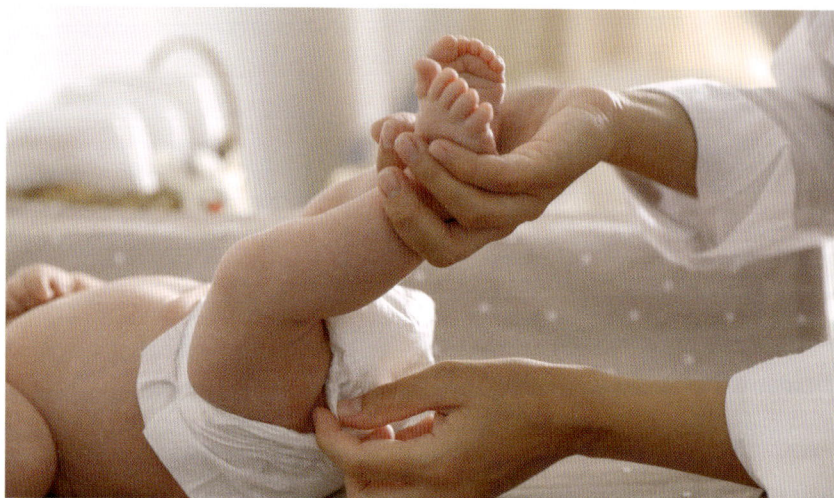

© New Africa/Adobe Stock

Diapering method—cloth versus disposable—and diapering brand may also make a difference. For example, many brands of disposable diapers use a chlorine bleaching process that produces toxic byproducts; "super-absorbent" diapers contain the same substance associated with toxic shock syndrome.[244] There is no regulatory requirement for diaper manufacturers to test their materials for hazardous chemicals.[245] If using disposables, choose brands that are chlorine-free, latex-free and free of dyes and fragrances, such as disposables made of bamboo.[246]

Many brands of easy-to-use cloth diapers are available. Washing cloth diapers in a mild, fragrance-free soap and adding an extra rinse with vinegar can help keep irritants that might lead to diaper rash away from baby's skin.

> " In 2020, tens of thousands of lawsuits forced Johnson & Johnson (J&J) to stop selling its well-known baby powder due to its inclusion of asbestos. "

Maternal Changes

"I looked on childrearing not only as a work of love and duty but as a profession that was fully interesting and challenging as any honorable profession in the world and one that demanded the best that I could bring to it."
— **Rose Kennedy,** *mother of former U.S. president John F. Kennedy*

Bringing an infant into the world changes a mother forever. After giving birth, the mother, her baby, and her husband or partner will adjust to their new life together. Sometimes, mothers may feel as if they have lost their identity; this feeling is normal. Self-awareness is key for adapting to the sometimes-overwhelming transition that all new mothers go through. Keeping mind, body, and spirit at ease can become an important if challenging everyday task. Healthy and happy children are the product of parents who take the initiative to find ways of cultivating their own personal growth.

It can be helpful for mothers to reflect on their nutritional, emotional, spiritual, and social habits:

- **Nutritional:** Is she limiting refined sugars and processed foods, and focusing on whole, nutrient-dense foods?
- **Emotional:** Is she feeling anxious or overwhelmed? Is she struggling with a situation at home or with a friend? Is a toxic relationship affecting her ability to release tension?
- **Spiritual:** Is she paying attention to what she absorbs from TV, social media, news channels, and other media? Is she mitigating stressful media consumption? Is she using healthy coping skills such as journaling, reading inspirational passages, or attending an adult or spiritual group?
- **Social:** Is she feeling isolated or having difficulty figuring out how to navigate a social life?

> *Healthy and happy children are the product of parents who take the initiative to find ways of cultivating their own personal growth.*

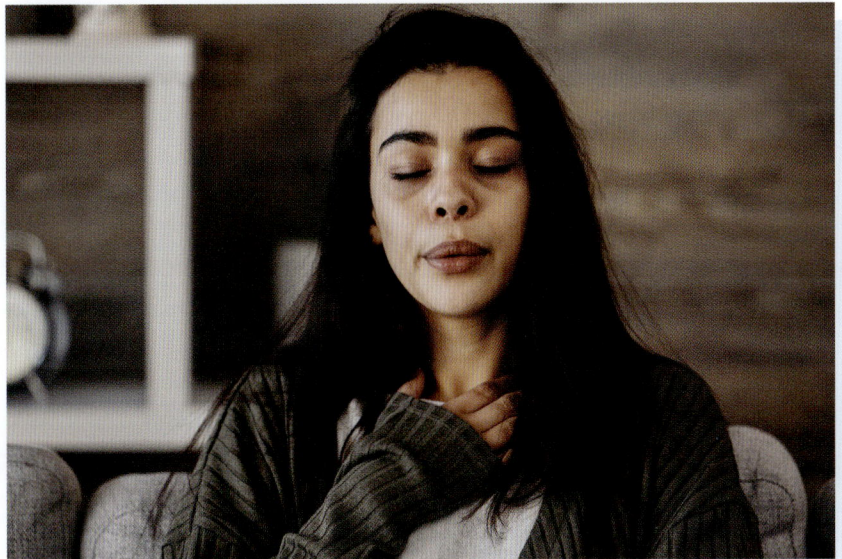

There are many resources to assist new mothers.[247] Social media can facilitate access to groups that provide social outlets for new mothers or new parents. Reaching out to friends, or meeting up with a group at a park or for coffee, or joining a fitness class in the community, are useful tools that may allow mothers to connect to others.

While caring for an infant, a mother initially may find it difficult to find time for herself, but as the baby grows and becomes more independent, she will find time to incorporate activities that refresh and provide positive energy. However, mothers often feel guilty about doing things for themselves. Society promotes the message that mothers should sacrifice themselves for their children. The truth is that mothers need to look after themselves, too—both for their children's sake and their own. When mothers constantly fulfill their children's needs but neglect their own, they may reach a point where they have no more to give. They can become exhausted, resentful, or angry because nobody is looking after them. Mothers may have to learn to ask for what they need. Moreover, if mothers always put their children first, they are modeling the behavior that their own needs don't matter; mothers who look after themselves present their children with a healthy role model.

Postpartum Depression

"Being a new mother is supposed to be the happiest time of your life, but postpartum depression and anxiety strip that away for a time. But trust that it will not last forever." — **Judy Dippel** (*professional author and speaker*)

A mother will go through many changes during and after a pregnancy. If a new mother feels empty, emotionless, or sad all or most of the time, or if she feels as if she doesn't love or care for her baby, it is likely postpartum depression. Researchers believe postpartum depression in a mother may have effects throughout childhood, including potentially contributing to developmental delays and learning problems,[248] and inhibiting mother–child bonding.[249]

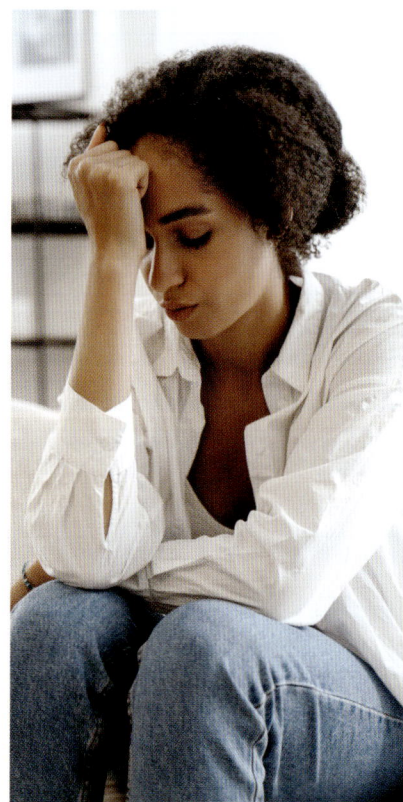

© Drobot Dean/Adobe Stock

> *When mothers constantly fulfill their children's needs but neglect their own, they may reach a point where they have no more to give.*

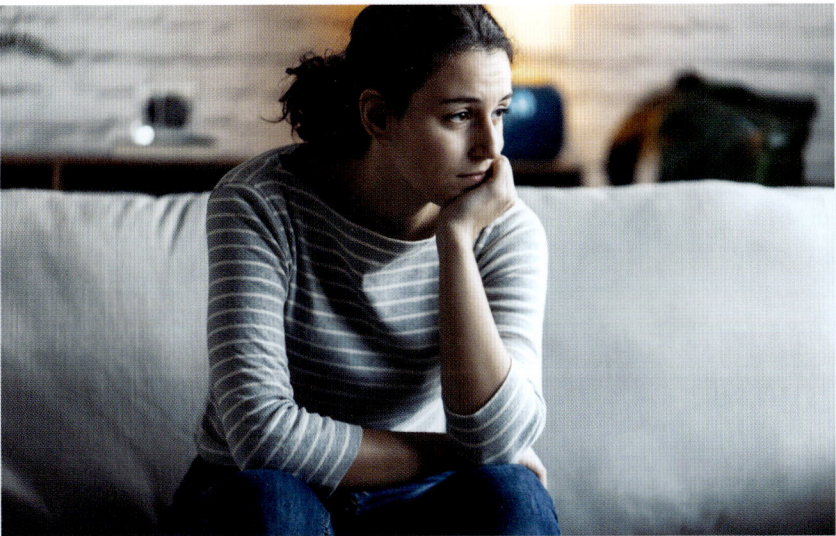

Postpartum Support International estimates that 15% to 20% of women experience "significant symptoms of depression or anxiety" after the birth of a child.[250] Approximately one out of nine women suffers from postpartum or postnatal depression. If the feelings persist for longer than two weeks during or after a pregnancy, clinicians recommend that mothers reach out for help. In some instances of postpartum depression, professionals may recommend treatments such as talk therapy or temporary pharmacologic intervention.

Hormonal changes can trigger symptoms of postpartum depression.[251] When a woman is pregnant, the female hormones estrogen and progesterone are the highest they'll ever be. In the first 24 hours after childbirth, these hormone levels quickly drop back to their normal, pre-pregnancy levels. Researchers believe this sudden change in hormonal levels—much more extreme than the changes that occur during menstruation—can lead to depression.

Levels of thyroid hormones also drop after a woman gives birth. The thyroid is a small gland in the neck that helps regulate how the body uses and stores energy from food. Low levels of thyroid hormones, too, may cause symptoms of depression. In women where there are reasons to suspect thyroid issues, hormone expert Dr. Jolene Brighten recommends working with a postpartum thyroid expert, who can order a thyroid lab panel and other relevant lab tests and review natural and medication treatment options.[252]

> " *Hormonal changes can trigger symptoms of postpartum depression.* "

During pregnancy, maternal zinc levels fall as copper levels rise, and zinc deficiency is another possible cause of postnatal depression.[253] Zinc, a trace mineral, has the second highest concentration in the brain of all transition metals (metals important to the chemistry of living systems). Research also links zinc deficiency to behavioral disturbances.[254]

Clinicians and researchers have found a lower zinc blood concentration in women with postpartum depression. Ellen Grant, a physician and medical gynecologist in the UK, has noted that a shortage of zinc, along with magnesium, in women prior to conception may cause infertility and recurrent miscarriages, also stating that years of pre-pregnancy hormonal contraceptive use will increase deficiencies of these minerals.[255] She adds that all of this is likely contributing to the "extremely high incidence" of postnatal depression, "with increased risk of long term adverse effects on child development." Further, "Deficiencies of trace elements like zinc, copper and magnesium have been implicated in various reproductive events like infertility, pregnancy wastage, congenital anomalies, pregnancy induced hypertension, placental abruption, premature rupture of membranes, stillbirths and low birth weight."

Untreated postpartum depression can affect a mother's ability to parent. She may struggle with low energy, mood swings, an inability to fully care for her baby, and maybe even a higher risk of suicide. Fortunately, help is available for depressed mothers. Postpartum Support International offers expert guidance, resources, and peer support group meetings.[256]

> *Untreated postpartum depression can affect a mother's ability to parent.*

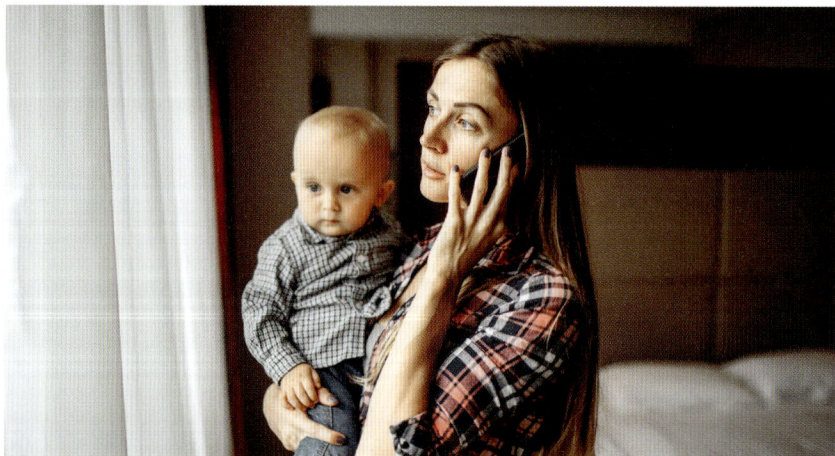

© Nomad_Soul/Adobe Stock

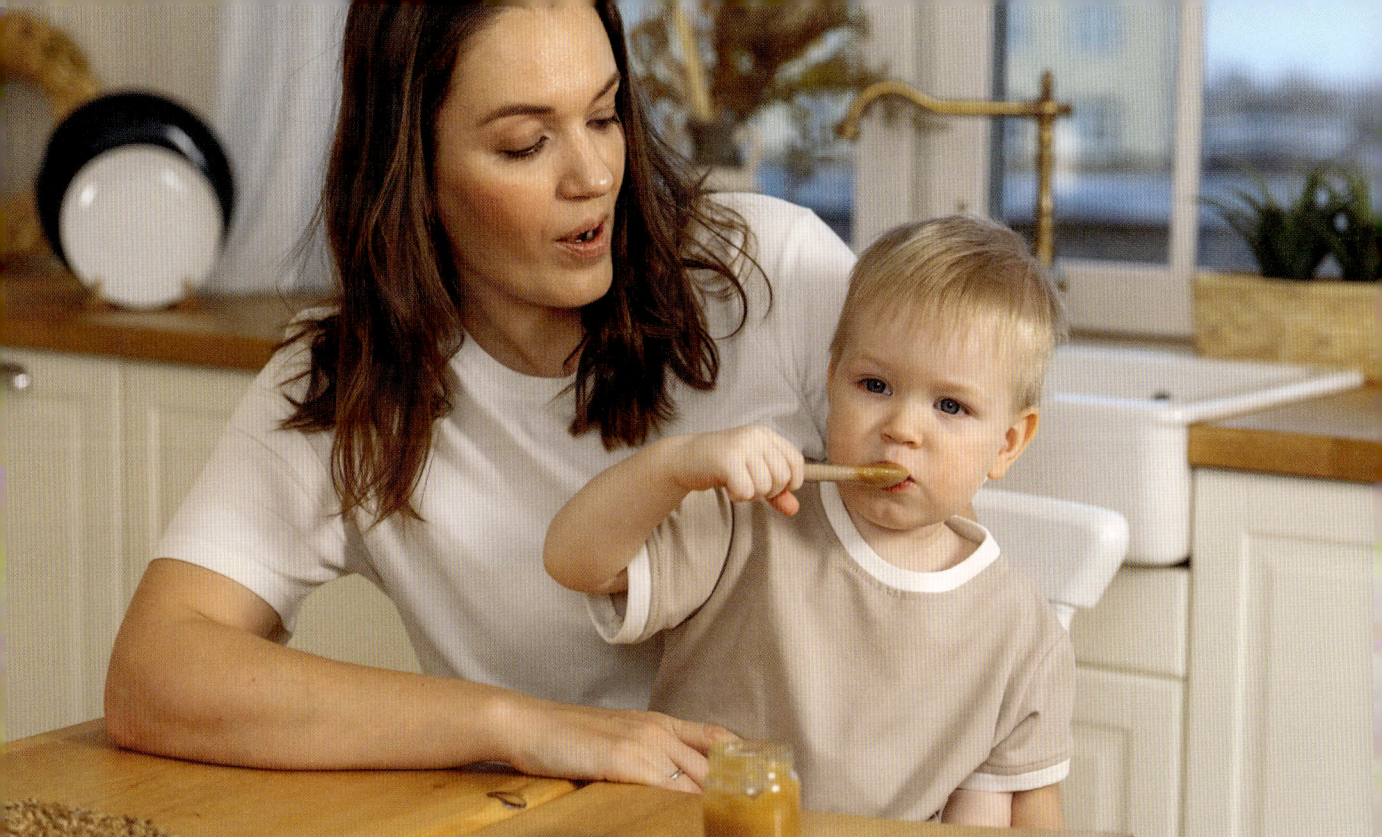

Chapter Five: The Solid Food Transition

"Let food be thy medicine, thy medicine shall be thy food." — **Hippocrates**

Parents should support their children with natural, unprocessed foods. Food is medicine—especially for a developing infant. The more processed a food is, the less nutritional value it has.

In this chapter, we will:

- Discuss how to approach the introduction of solid foods
- Describe how to watch for possible allergic reactions

Introducing Solid Food

There is widespread agreement that sometime between the fourth and sixth months is the optimal time to introduce solid foods; in combination with solid foods, breastfeeding (or homemade formula) can then continue for as long as mother and baby wish. Most organizations do not recommend

> *There is widespread agreement that sometime between the fourth and sixth months is the optimal time to introduce solid foods.*

introducing solid foods before four months of age due to the risk of gastrointestinal problems and allergies. Sally Fallon Morell of the Weston A. Price Foundation points to research indicating that introducing solids in the four- to six-month window may, in fact, "result in the lowest allergy risk."[257] Morell also emphasizes:

> "There is no age at which baby is growing faster—and forming more connections in the brain—than the age from zero to one. This is not the time to be casual about feeding your baby—because food before one matters a ton!"[258]

Morell disputes the notion that when babies push food back out, it means they are "not ready" or "not hungry," instead noting that babies are simply "learning how to eat." They may also subsequently appreciate a food that they initially reject.

Because of infants' rapid growth and development, Morell insists that nutrient density is as or more important for little ones as for adults. Infants' immature digestive systems are poorly equipped to handle carbohydrates but can supply the enzymes needed to digest fats and proteins. She takes issue with the suggestion to let babies play with items like raw vegetables or extruded rice cakes and says, "above all, babies need animal fats":

> "[Animal fats] are critical for growth, hormone production and indeed practically all functions in the body, right down to the mitochondria. Animal fats provide cholesterol for neurological development; arachidonic acid for healthy skin, brains and digestion; and fat-soluble vitamins needed for just about everything, including iron assimilation and hormone production."

> **Because of infants' rapid growth and development, Morell insists that nutrient density is as or more important for little ones as for adults.**

© Brebca/Adobe Stock

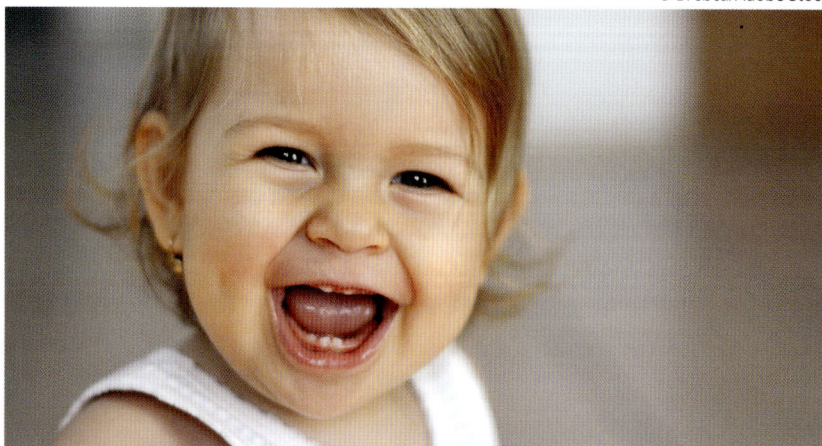

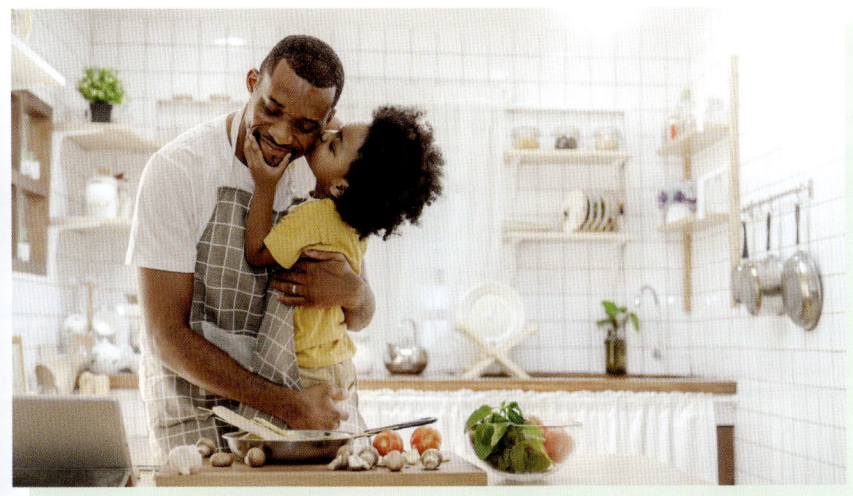

Morell advises starting with homemade foods that parents have puréed, ground up, or finely minced. (Store-bought baby foods often contain additives and other undesirable ingredients, and frequently come in phthalate-laden plastic containers or aluminum-lined packaging.) Morell also emphasizes the critical importance of salt for infant digestion and brain development, criticizing those who would deprive babies of magnesium, trace minerals, and sodium by putting them on a low-salt diet.

Organic whole foods support optimal development and strong endocrine and immune systems.[259] Organic foods and pastured meats contain fewer pesticides and heavy metals, no antibiotics or synthetic hormones, and healthy fats and healthy antioxidants.[260]

From a nutrient-density standpoint, says Morell, there are two ideal first foods, which can start as early as four months of age:

- Soft or runny egg yolks from pastured hens (either scooped out of a whole egg boiled for three and a half minutes, or in the form of a runny yolk taken from a fried egg, with a pinch of salt added), building up from half a teaspoon (if baby seems to react poorly, parents can wait a couple of weeks and then try again)

- Liver puréed with a little salt, broth, and butter or cream ("baby paté"), obtained from healthy animals that spend their lives on pasture or (as the next best choice) from organically raised animals[261]

> *Organic foods and pastured meats contain fewer pesticides and heavy metals, no antibiotics or synthetic hormones, and healthy fats and healthy antioxidants.*

Around six to eight months, parents can add:

- Red meat, fish, or dark chicken puréed "with water, bone broth, raw milk or cream, and always with added fat, especially butter"
- Well-cooked fruit and vegetables, puréed or mashed with cream or butter
- Creamed soups
- Custards

Over time, babies can progress to finger foods cut into small pieces, such as:

- Ripe banana pieces (or banana mashed with a little cream and a pinch of salt)
- Organic cheese (preferably raw rather than pasteurized)
- Bits of natural bacon
- Dried anchovies or fish eggs

Morell cautions against introducing harder-to-digest foods until a baby is at least one year old. Difficult-to-digest foods include grains, egg whites, and raw fruits and vegetables. One suggestion for introducing whole eggs is to scramble them with extra yolks and cream. As for grains, parents should cook them well after making them more digestible by soaking them overnight in water with a small amount of lemon juice, vinegar, yogurt, or kefir. A high-quality sourdough bread "spread thickly with butter" can also enter the repertoire at this time.

The Weston A. Price Foundation website offers many other practical suggestions about when and how to feed babies.[262]

> *Over time, babies can progress to finger foods cut into small pieces.*

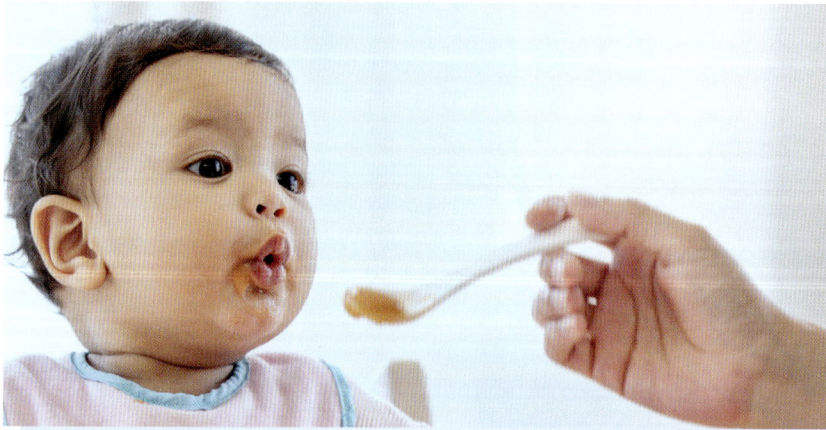

© Jade Maas/peopleimages.com/Adobe Stock

Food Reactions and Food Allergies

When introducing new foods, it is best to add new foods every five to seven days. Adding the new food at breakfast time allows parents to watch for any reactions during the day. Any food that an infant has had without any reaction for five to seven days is generally safe to give in combination with other safe foods that the infant can tolerate.

Parents can watch for negative reactions that sometimes follow the introduction of new foods:[263]

- Redness around the mouth
- Bloating, gas
- Frequent spitting up
- Nasal or chest congestion
- Constipation
- Diarrhea
- Eczema-like skin rash
- Fussiness, irritability
- Difficulty sleeping

An estimated 1 in 12 children has food allergies,[264] and the prevalence of pediatric food allergies has risen by at least 50% since the late 1990s.[265] A study conducted for the decade-long period from 2005 to 2014 showed that pediatric emergency department visits for food-related anaphylaxis increased by 214%, with the highest rates in infants and toddlers.[266] Over roughly the same period, an analysis of tens of billions of private health insurance claims for children and adults showed that claims with diagnoses of food anaphylaxis (two-thirds of which were for children) rose by 377%, with peanut allergies topping the list.[267] Other leading food allergens include pasteurized cow's milk (and related dairy products), egg whites, tree nuts, sesame seeds, shellfish and fish, wheat/gluten, and soy, as well as unnatural ingredients like preservatives, food additives, and monosodium glutamate (MSG). MSG is present not just in many processed foods but also as a stabilizer in some vaccines such as the chickenpox (varicella) and measles-mumps-rubella-varicella (MMRV) vaccines.[268]

> *An estimated 1 in 12 children has food allergies, and the prevalence of pediatric food allergies has risen by at least 50% since the late 1990s.*

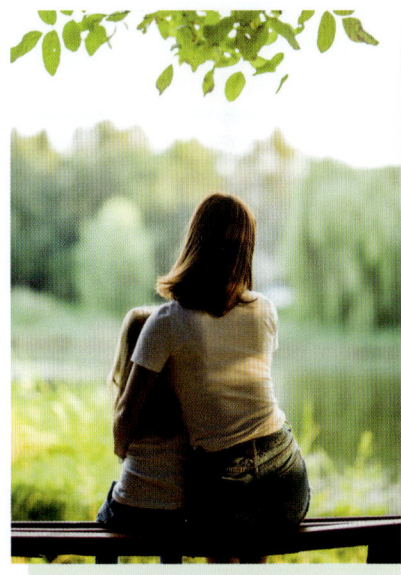

© F8\Support Ukraine/Adobe Stock

Mainstream medicine declares itself baffled as to the causes of the food allergy epidemic, but experiments dating back over a century suggest that the allergies are largely iatrogenic—and point to medical injections and injected vaccines, in particular, as likely culprits.[269] The major expansion of the childhood vaccine schedule since the late 1980s, the day-of-birth hepatitis B vaccines and vitamin K shots, the widespread use of immune-dysregulating aluminum adjuvants,[270] and changes in vaccine technology are all factors that can explain the "immunoexcitotoxic" cascade that is manifesting in the form of food allergies and other disorders such as autism.[271,272] As the authors of a 2016 study summed up:

> "The era of food allergy began with the post-millennial generation, the same faction who received new immunizations during early childhood. Many of these vaccines contain alum, an adjuvant known to induce allergic phenotypes." [273]

In *The Peanut Allergy Epidemic: What's Causing it and How to Stop It*, author Heather Fraser drew attention to a 1991 paper that put forth the plausible view of allergy as a form of immunological defense against certain toxins.[274,275] From this perspective, allergy symptoms such as vomiting, sneezing, and decreased blood pressure are logical bodily responses designed to expel toxic substances—such as those present in vaccines—or slow their circulation in the body.

> *Allergy symptoms such as vomiting, sneezing, and decreased blood pressure are logical bodily responses designed to expel toxic substances.*

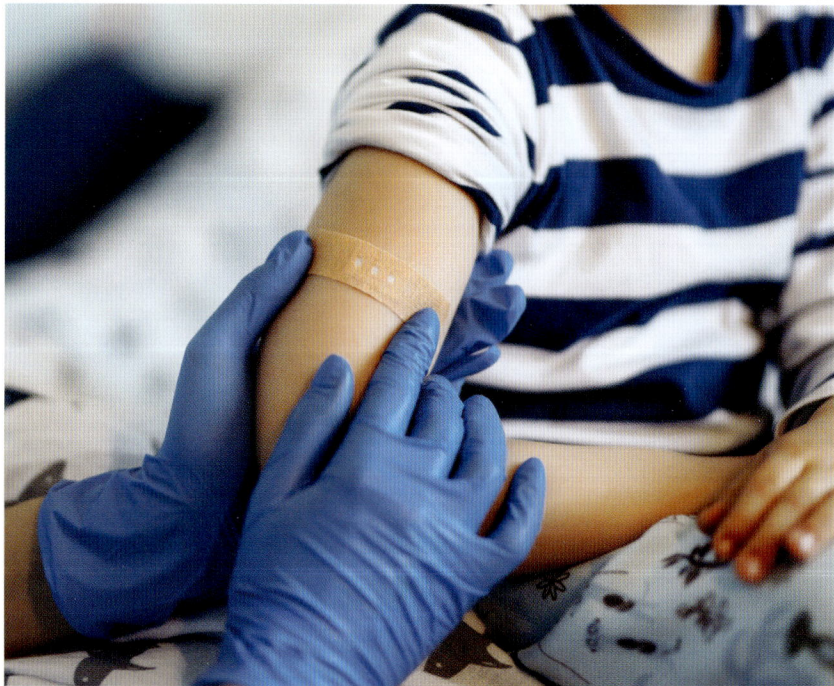

© maxbelchenko/Adobe Stock

As noted in the preceding chapter, studies comparing the health of vaccinated and unvaccinated children and adults consistently show that vaccination increases the likelihood of allergies and related conditions like eczema and asthma.[276] Although vaccines are not the sole trigger for the development of food allergies, parents who wish to minimize their babies' risks would do well to understand the probable relationship.

Other factors linked to childhood food allergies—and to skin rashes, hay fever, and asthma—include early-life exposure to antibiotics and antacids prescribed for reflux;[277] exposure to tobacco smoke and mold (as well as cockroaches and mites);[278] and exposure to GMO ingredients,[279] glyphosate and other pesticides.[280] On the other hand, many studies point to farm and rural environments as protective against allergies, with effects continuing into young adulthood.[281] Specific protective factors associated with those environments include exposure to livestock and their fodder and consumption of raw milk.[282,283]

Avoiding the toxic exposures that contribute to the development of allergies and other allergic conditions is the best prevention. If allergies develop, parents may wish to familiarize themselves with the range of options available. Conventional medicine is likely to advise over-the-counter antihistamines like Benadryl but may not mention the drug's strong sedative effects or conversely, its tendency to induce hyperactivity in 10% to 15% of children.[284] For those susceptible to anaphylactic reactions, doctors recommend having epinephrine (an "EpiPen") on hand, though EpiPens are expensive and prone to regular recalls.[285]

Many non-drug approaches to managing and healing allergies are available, including making dietary changes (including strictly avoiding GMOs and glyphosate-exposed ingredients), increasing intake of probiotics or fermented foods, and exploring natural alternatives such as herbal remedies, homeopathy, and acupuncture.

> *Avoiding the toxic exposures that contribute to the development of allergies and other allergic conditions is the best prevention.*

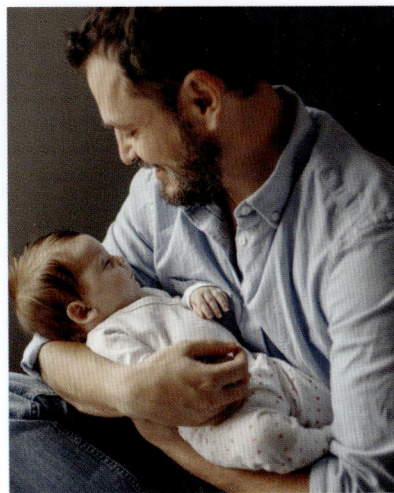

© anoushkatoronto/Adobe Stock

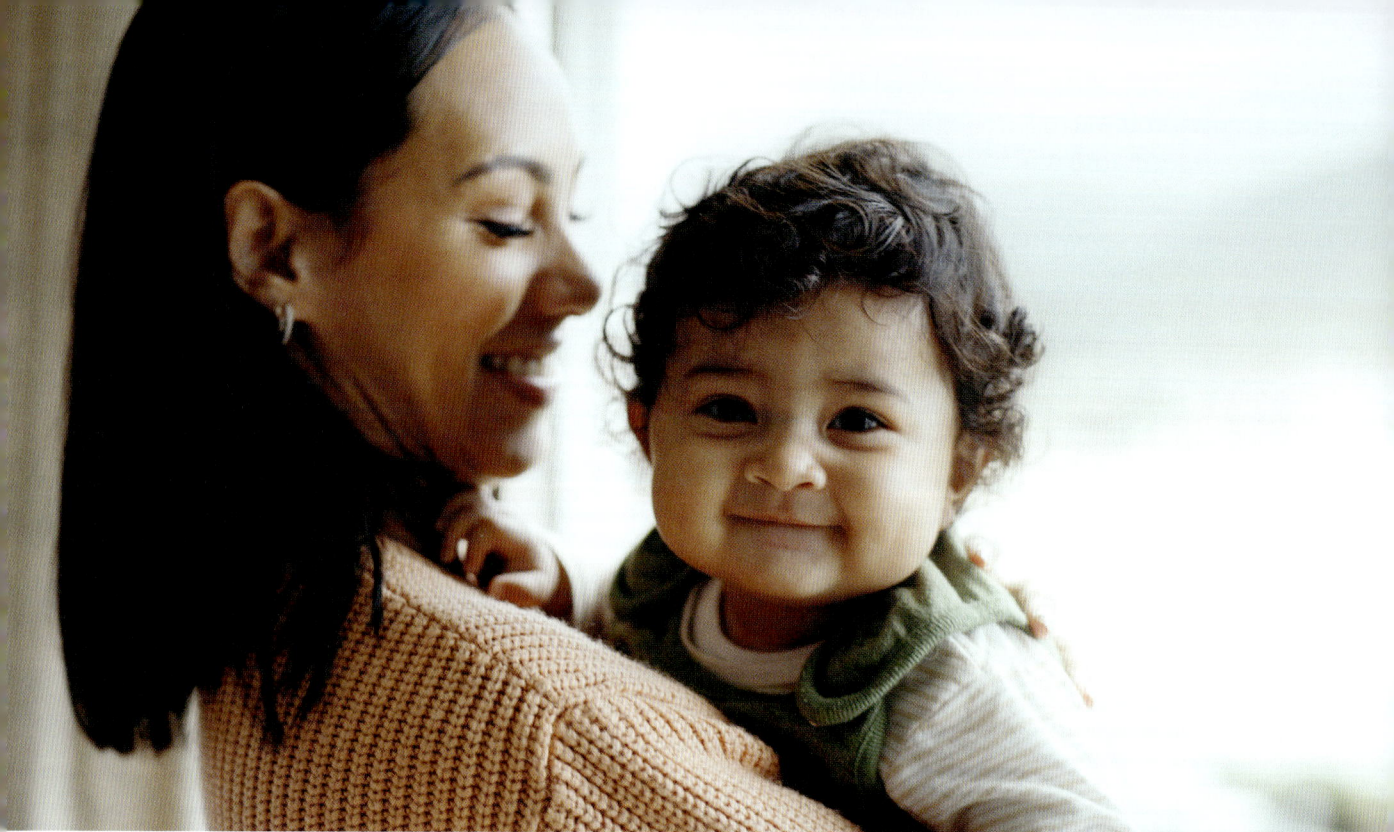

Chapter Six: Developmental Milestones

"Learning springs naturally in newborn babies and young children. Though you do not need to teach your baby how to see, you can place him in interesting and colorful environments. We do not need to teach him how to feel, but we can offer him new things to touch and explore. Your newborn baby's interests and curiosity in people and the world are already there, inside him. They are in-built, as this is with other senses. He just needs you to offer him the right opportunities and he will develop at his own inner pace."
— **John Thomson et al.,** *Natural Childbirth* **(1995)**

From the very beginning, a baby responds to and also initiates interactions with people and responds to various types of attention. Parents and babies share control of their conversations and negotiate an exchange that includes facial expressions such as smiling and laughing.

What is taking place between parent and baby is rather like the performance of a pair of highly practiced dancers.

What is taking place between parent and baby is rather like the performance of a pair of highly practiced dancers.

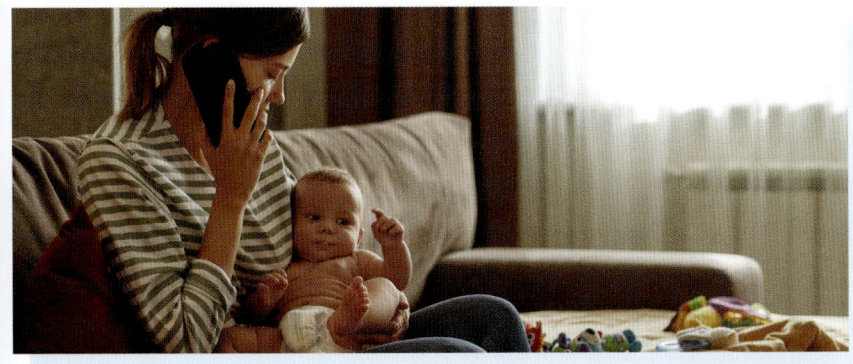

Unfortunately, exposure to "ubiquitous but insidious" environmental toxins can threaten babies' healthy development, and "too little has been done to protect [them]."[286] (For more details on environmental toxins, see Chapter Seven.) The prevalence of developmental delays and disabilities has been increasing steadily since the 1990s; a government study published in 2019 concluded that the percentage of children diagnosed with a developmental disability increased significantly between 2009 and 2017, resulting in a growing population of children (one in six) with one or more developmental disabilities.[287] Among children with any disability, cognitive difficulties are the most common type, affecting 4.4% of children ages 5–17 according to the U.S. Census Bureau.[288] The CDC's most recent estimate of autism prevalence, for surveillance year 2018, is that 1 in 44 eight-year-olds in the U.S. had received an autism spectrum disorder diagnosis.[289]

Environmental toxins like lead and fluoride are by now well-documented causes of cognitive and behavioral problems in children,[290,291] but in addition, vaccines demand attention as a probable culprit, particularly given that the dramatic surge in developmental disabilities began around the same time that the CDC started expanding the types and total number of vaccines on the childhood vaccine schedule.[292]

In this chapter, we will:

- Describe parent-child communication as a rewarding process of teaching and learning

- Review how speech begins

- Discuss how parents can anticipate and support their children's needs

- Outline typical growth and development milestones and note the CDC's recent changes to those milestones

- Describe types of developmental delays

- Discuss the likely association of vaccination and developmental delays

> *The prevalence of developmental delays and disabilities has been increasing steadily since the 1990s.*

Teaching and Learning: The Joy of Communication

In their enduring 1995 book, *Natural Childhood*, John Thomson and co-authors describe many ways that parents can support their developing child. They note that although nobody teaches parents how to play face games with their baby, all parents instinctively initiate and join in such activities with great sensitivity. Parents may raise the pitch of their voice, slow down the rhythm of their speech, or add a sing-song quality, speaking in 5- to 15-second intervals. This combination of timing and sound is ideal for holding a baby's brief attention span, and resonates with the baby's inbuilt rhythm.

Babies are sensitive to parents' responses from the moment of birth. Researchers call this process "attunement,"[293] and they believe that it is a critical step in the process of a baby learning to speak.[294] As babies' needs become more complex, they will be motivated to start using words. If they are developing normally, they will acquire language as they need it.

Many of the interactions between babies and their parents take place intuitively. Babies behave spontaneously in the only way they know how, and their parents respond intuitively. As described in *Natural Childhood*:

"As your baby grows and changes you adapt your behavior to suit him. Face games turn into body games and body games develop into nursery rhymes, without anyone teaching you to do it. The pattern of a healthy relationship is there right from the start. What is important is that it is maintained and can develop and flourish. An important aspect of the relationship between parent and child is teaching and learning. Parents don't think of themselves and their children as teachers and students but teaching and learning go on between them all the time."

> **Although nobody teaches parents how to play face games with their baby, all parents instinctively initiate and join in such activities with great sensitivity.**

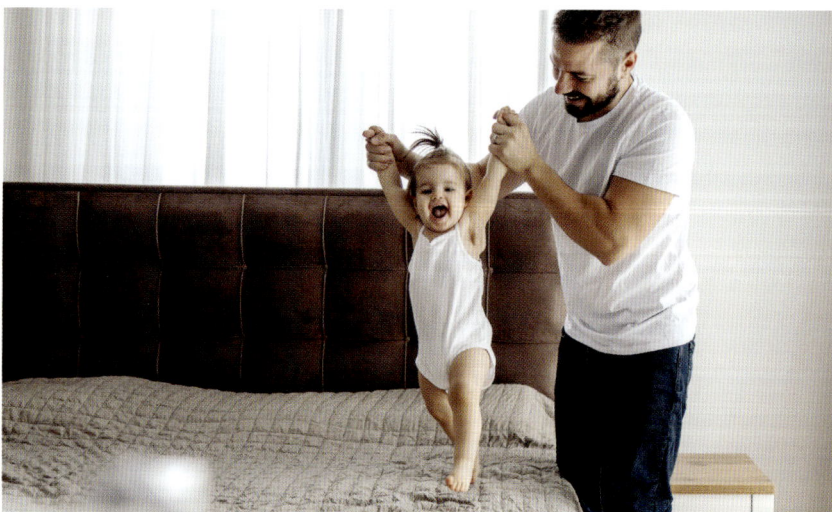

© Dusan Petkovic/Adobe Stock

Unfortunately, some parents have lost touch with this innate human sense and rely on experts who "know best" and tell parents what their child ought to be doing when, or advise remedial actions if they view the child as a "late developer." Parents may feel great pressure for their child to achieve and may be tempted to push the child at too fast a pace. This may appear to reap rewards in the short term, but it is likely to cause tensions in the end. Parents must trust themselves as to what their baby needs.

Anticipating and Responding to a Child's Needs

Children have three broad categories of essential needs:

- Food, warmth, exercise, and sleep
- Love and a sense of belonging
- Opportunities to explore, question, experience, and learn

Parents cannot know what goes on inside their child's head; they can only guess what the child is thinking and feeling through their words and actions. As a young child explores and learns, some needs will merely require the parents to be observers, while others will require parental participation. The parents' role is to sense, as best as they can, what their child needs and when.

A child "works" all day and every day, but at any given moment, all a parent may need to do is just acknowledge what the child is learning about life. As the authors of *Natural Childhood* put it, children are "learning all the time. For there is no distinction between learning and playing. There is no need to set up special learning opportunities for a child."

> *Parents must trust themselves as to what their baby needs.*

© bernardbodo/Adobe Stock

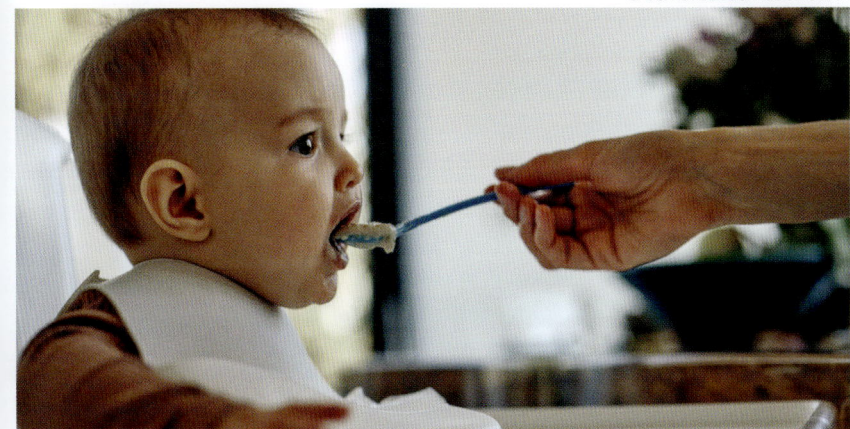

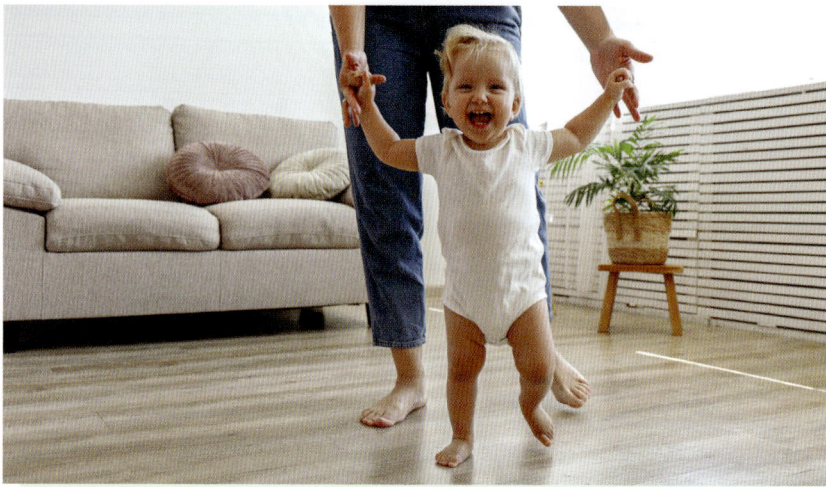
© Evrymmnt/Adobe Stock

As human beings, we learn best when we feel good about ourselves. If we are upset, we get distracted, and we may need to take time to resolve our upset before being able to concentrate fully on our work. It is the same for a child. When children are upset, they may not be able to learn. Helping a child deal with whatever is on their mind will help them get back to the task at hand.

Every moment is an opportunity for a child to learn, but learning is also a process. When a child approaches a new task, they are likely to find it difficult, and it may take them many weeks to master it. For example, learning to walk may proceed as a series of attempts to stand upright, move one foot in front of the other, and take a few steps—punctuated by moments of falling over or screaming with frustration—before the child finally is able to walk unaided. Perseverance brings success. Along the way, the child will benefit from active parental encouragement (see "How Parents Can Help Children Learn, Grow, and Develop"). When a parent says, "You can do it," that affirmation guides the child toward success and helps them appreciate their achievements. This attitude will affect their approach to every task throughout their life, helping them develop confidence in their ability to succeed.

> *Every moment is an opportunity for a child to learn, but learning is also a process.*

Children must learn through their own successes and mistakes. As much as parents might like to protect their children from life's hard knocks, they cannot, and it is important that they don't. Such experiences are an essential part of growing up.

How Parents Can Help Children Learn, Grow, and Develop

- Listen to the child's ideas.
- Point out their achievements.
- Think through difficult situations with them.
- Let them learn from their mistakes.
- Make time for them.
- Stop telling them what to do.
- Stop telling them what they are doing wrong.

Children Set the Pace

Children learn at their own pace. They will learn to speak when they feel the need to communicate ideas to others. They will learn to walk when crawling or shuffling fails to give them enough mobility. Parents who are desperate for a child to learn a particular skill at a particular time may even find that their urging backfires, making it less likely that the child will want to learn it. Children have invisible antennae that pick up their parents' unexpressed wishes, and that does influence their behavior!

> *Children learn at their own pace. They will learn to speak when they feel the need to communicate ideas to others.*

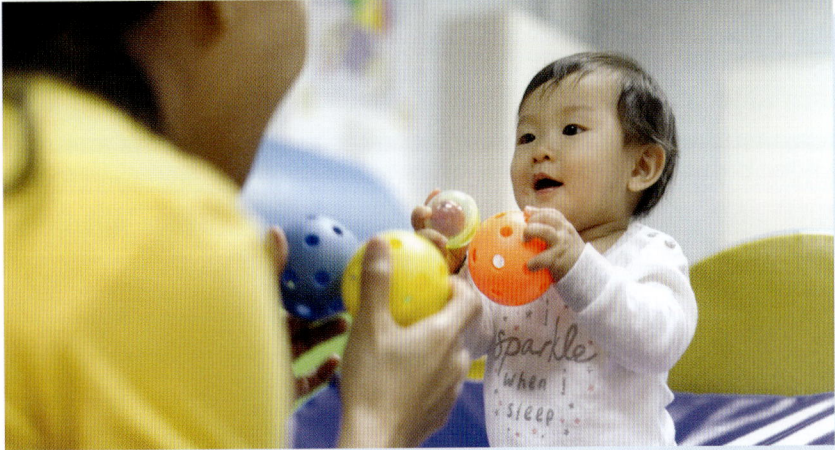

© Kawee/Adobe Stock

Adults sometimes find it hard to hold back. When they offer suggestions as to how a child could do something better, the child may be hurt and might even tell the parents to "leave them alone." That said, the ability to give a child attention without interfering is a helpful skill to cultivate.

As parents observe the learning in which their child is engaged, they may be able to give appropriate assistance, but in general, children need to explore and experience life. At the same time, children want the security of boundaries. As parents communicate what is and is not okay, the boundaries should be flexible enough not to interfere with a child's need to experience life, yet firm enough to guide a child who does not yet have a realistic sense of their own abilities and limitations. Ultimately, parents' job is to let their child's curiosity and desire to learn unfold and develop in a healthy way, while ensuring that the child does not put themselves in harm's way (such as pulling a plastic bag over their head in the name of "exploration") and only suffers the knocks and bruises that inevitably accompany day-to-day life.

A loving presence is invaluable. There will be times when a child will play on their own, but when parents try to slip away unnoticed, the child may demand that the parent stay. Just because a child does not constantly turn to a parent for reassurance and encouragement does not mean that the child does not want and need parental attention and presence.

If a child is playing quietly, parents may consider merely sitting with them quietly. If the child is dancing, a parent may try moving with them. Society conditions adults to believe that they know best because of their greater knowledge and experience, and they often find it hard to let the child take the lead. However, children have a lot to teach their parents and can offer many new perspectives on life if parents are open to receiving them.

It is said that human beings' need to love is greater than the need to be loved. A child provides the opportunity to love nonstop, awakening a depth of loving and seeking a parent's unconditional love in return.

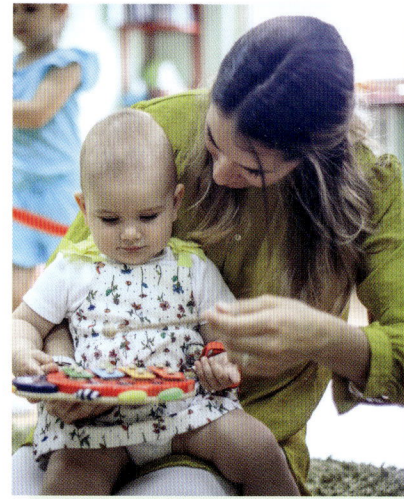

© liderina/Adobe Stock

> **A child provides the opportunity to love nonstop, awakening a depth of loving and seeking a parent's unconditional love in return.**

Developmental Milestones

For many years, milestones for child development were those set out in the Appendix, which summarizes typical growth and development from infancy through toddlerhood.[295]

Physical and Motor Development

Babies learn every day and experience rapid development. Some of baby's first milestones involve physical and motor development. Physical development means growth in height, increase in weight, change of shape, and the completion of the structures of the different organs of the body. It also implies increased control over the body, and the ability to move the limbs, use the hands, coordinate hand and eye movements, and stand, run, and jump. An early motor milestone is the baby's ability to hold their head up without support. Babies generally reach this milestone between *two and four months* of age.

Also between *two and four months*, a baby will be able to push up with his arms when lying on his stomach. "Tummy time" helps strengthen the upper body and neck muscles that a baby needs to sit up. Allowing a two-month-old baby to have supervised tummy time at least three times per day for several minutes each time will help encourage the baby to meet this milestone.

A baby may start rolling over as early as *four months* of age. The baby may start by rocking side to side, which is the motion that is fundamental to rolling over. Once babies master rolling over from tummy to back, they will master rolling from back to tummy. At four to six months old, a baby should typically roll over in both directions. To encourage rolling over, parents can place babies on a blanket on the floor with a toy or book near them that they can reach toward with their arms.

> " An early motor milestone is the baby's ability to hold their head up without support. "

© Prostock-studio/Adobe Stock

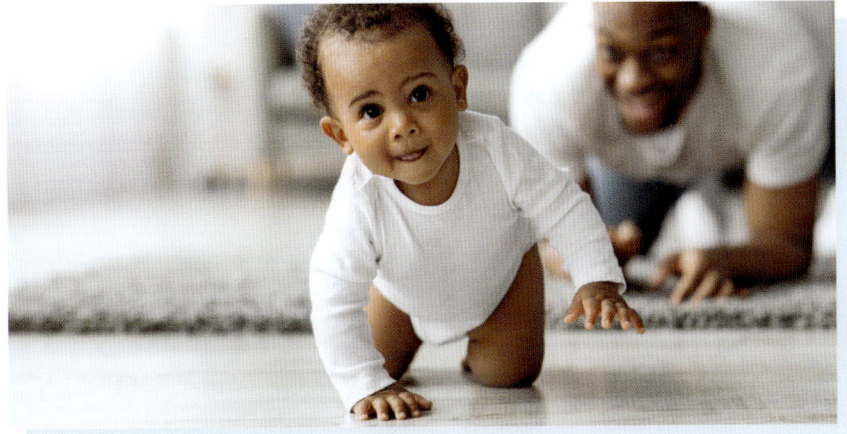

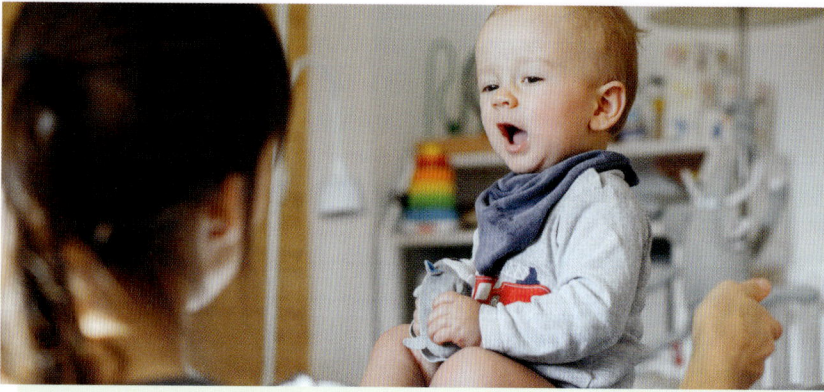

© Iryna/Adobe Stock

At around *six months*, babies will have developed enough upper body strength to begin to sit up unsupported. Parents can help babies sit up by supporting them with pillows.

At *nine months*, a baby should be able to sit well and be able to get out of a sitting position with minimal help.

At *12 months*, a baby should be able to get into a sitting position without help.

Speech and Early Play

We do not inherit our language. Rather, a newborn baby has the potential to acquire any of the 6,000 languages that humanity speaks. A baby placed among speakers of one or more languages will acquire that language or those languages. Newborns have the ability to vocalize and also to respond to language and have an inborn capacity to grasp the structure basic to all languages.

A child's speaking ability begins with coos, gurgles, and babbling. At first, certain vowel-like sounds will emerge, followed by sounds of consonants. After just six weeks, a child will be able to repeat strings of sounds continually. Babies endlessly rehearse, are aware of, and enjoy rhythms, changes of pitch, and sound groups. Every vowel and consonant has a special quality. This is why nursery rhymes are so enjoyable for children. Their meaning can be strange, but their sounds are magical. For the child, words have magic and power.

A young child will combine gestures of reaching, pointing, and pushing away with sounds that communicate their needs, thoughts, and feelings. With these actions and sounds, they are deliberately trying to attract another person's interest and get them to act in the way they want. In essence, they are communicating without words.

A newborn baby has the potential to acquire any of the 6,000 languages that humanity speaks.

By about *two months* of age, the communication between baby and parents will have developed into face games involving expressions and gestures, with each playing a part.

When a baby is around *five months old*, parents may start to sing action songs and nursery rhymes intuitively. Even though babies cannot yet sing the words, they can learn actions and respond to the rhythms. They are not just imitating their parents; they are also following the rhyme and coordinating their hand and body movements in response.

Around *six months* of age, babies begin babbling as they get better at controlling their vowel sounds and the pitch and quality of their expressions. They have reached a point where they want to communicate. Also at six months, they can play a game in which they follow instructions, such as putting wooden dolls into a toy truck and taking them out again.

At around *nine months*, another significant development takes place. For the last few months, the infant has been able to either play with an object or interact in person-to-person games, but now they learn to do both at the same time.

As a child becomes more mobile, their world expands. Children start to learn names for people, objects, and actions. They can reach and handle many new objects, and they need to be able to talk about these new activities. From this point on, their communication will increase rapidly from baby language, which only their own family understands, to child language, which others can understand.

To help children learn language and achieve expected speech and language milestones, parents should:

- Talk, read, and play with their children
- Listen and respond to what a child says
- Talk with children in the language that they are most comfortable using
- Teach a child to speak another language if the parents speak one
- Talk about what they do and what their children do during the day
- Use a lot of different words
- Use longer sentences as the child gets older
- Encourage the child to play with other children

Around six months of age, babies begin babbling as they get better at controlling their vowel sounds and the pitch and quality of their expressions.

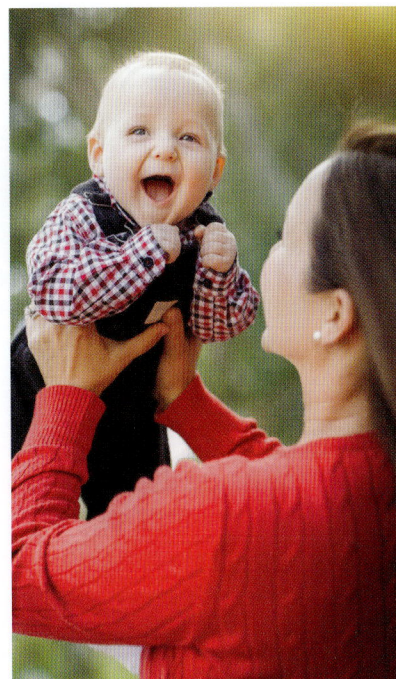

© Andy Dean/Adobe Stock

Crawling

Experts at Michigan State University (MSU) have identified as "prerequisites" for children to begin crawling the ability "to lift their head off the ground, to support their upper-body with their arms, to get their knees underneath them and being stable on all fours."[296] Around six months old, children will get into this position and just rock back and forth on hands and knees. This is a building block to crawling. As a child rocks, he may start to crawl backward before moving forward. By seven to 10 months old, a baby will begin to crawl. The MSU experts note the importance of crawling taking place on hands and knees with a cross-body pattern—"meaning the right arm and left leg go forward together"—that is different from belly crawling or scooting.

Crawling is important for proper brain development as well as for increasing bone and muscle strength and building future motor skills. The MSU researchers note that crawling is usually "a result of reaching for a toy that [babies] can't quite get to, and then they fall toward their outstretched hand. After they fall forward they realize they just moved closer to the object that they want."

Further discussing the importance of crawling, the MSU authors explain:

"As children crawl their brain is making more and more connections. Each connection is a solution to a problem that they have solved by, and with crawling. The more they crawl the more streamlined these connections become and the more automatic the skill becomes. Crawling provides them an opportunity to explore their environment. Before the skill becomes automatic, the child is using a lot of their brain just to move, and figure out what is going on and how to achieve this great feat of independent movement. You should be able to see this skill becoming more automatic as their speed increases from very slow, to getting-into-everything, fast!"

> *By seven to 10 months old, a baby will begin to crawl.*

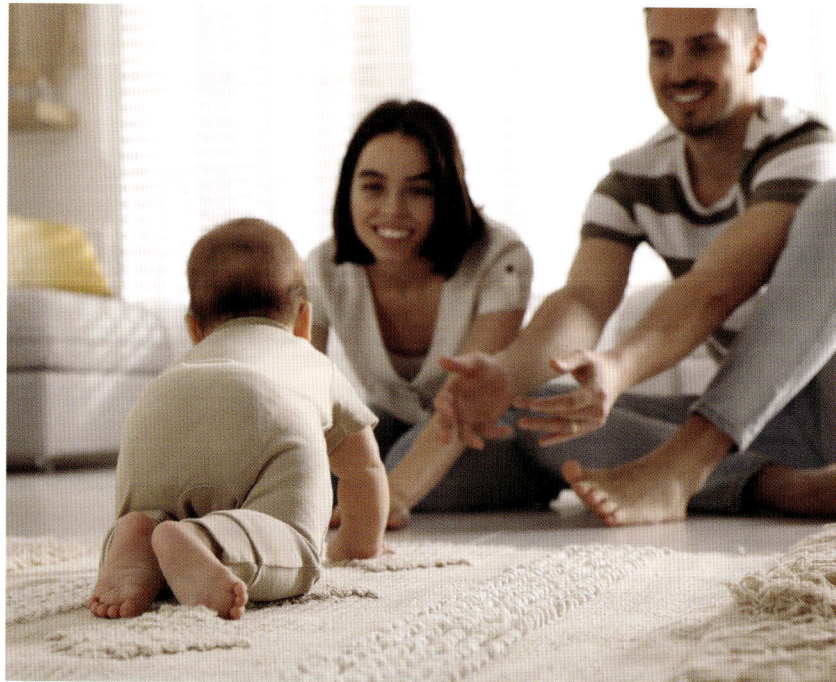

As crawling promotes the development of cognitive skills, children learn to locate objects by sight or touch. The MSU authors cite a study showing that children who had achieved hands-and-knees crawling could find a toy that had been hidden more often than children not crawling on hands and knees. They noted, "This was true no matter where in the room the child started looking for the toy," demonstrating crawling's important role in the development of both spatial and cognitive skills.

The MSU authors also emphasize another benefit of crawling: "a more flexible memory when learning new skills." They describe a study that compared children who were crawling with those not crawling, testing how well the children remembered a new skill taught to them after the researchers changed the environment. The former group "showed greater memory retention when tested in both the same and different settings." In other words, "Children who were not crawling needed the same stimuli and setting … to show retention of a skill, whereas children who were crawling were able to show skills where either the stimuli or the setting were different."

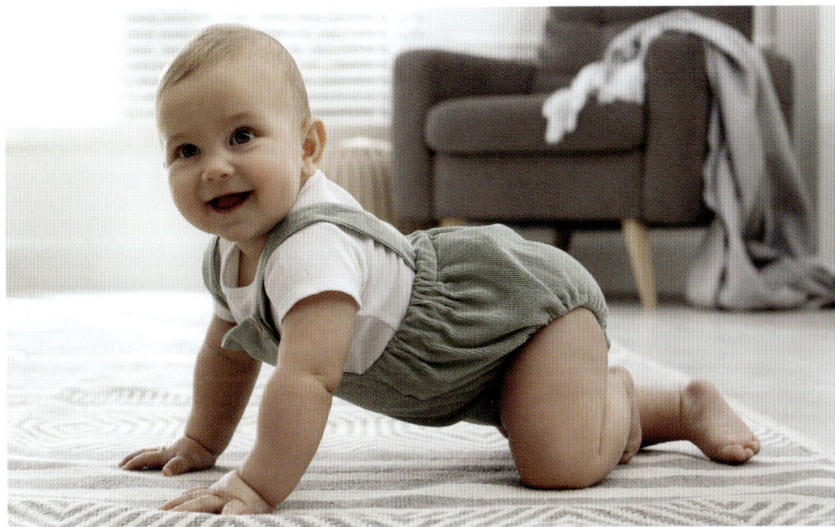

© New Africa/Adobe Stock

To support a child learning to crawl, parents should allow their baby to play on the floor in a safe area away from stairs. They can place favorite toys just out of reach as baby rocks back and forth, encouraging baby to reach for their toy.

Developmental Delays and the 2022 Revised Developmental Milestones

In February 2022, the CDC and AAP jointly revised the pediatric developmental milestones—for the first time since 2004—in the "Learn the Signs, Act Early" program.[297] This program, designed to help parents identify developmental delays in their children, includes milestone "checklists" or "markers."[298]

> 66
> *To support a child learning to crawl, parents should allow their baby to play on the floor in a safe area away from stairs.*
> 99

One of the organizations' stated reasons for modifying the milestones were concerns about the "wait-and-see approach" commonly employed by doctors and parents, which some experts believe causes delays in diagnosis of problems. Many times, pediatricians tell parents to "wait and see" because the child is too young to be diagnosed with a cognitive disorder. In some circumstances, it may be appropriate to merely monitor a child, but often this "wait-and-see" approach causes delays in appropriate evaluation.

CDC authors explained their revisions in a February 2022 article published in *Pediatrics*:

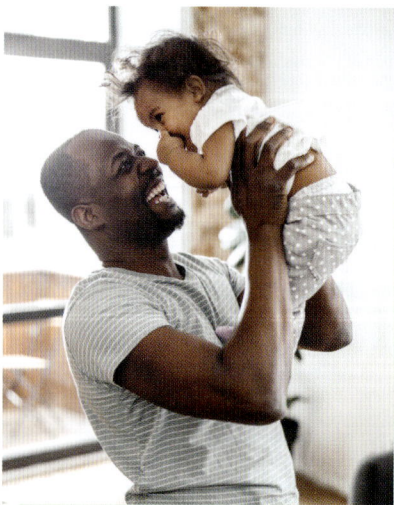

© Yakobchuk/Adobe Stock

"Subject matter experts identified by the AAP established 11 criteria for CDC milestone checklists, including using milestones most children (>75%) would be expected to achieve by specific health supervision visit ages and those that are easily observed in natural settings. A database of normative data for individual milestones, common screening and evaluation tools, and published clinical opinion was created to inform revisions. Application of the criteria established by the AAP working group and adding milestones for the 15- and 30-month health supervision visits resulted in a 26.4% reduction and 40.9% replacement of previous CDC milestones. One third of the retained milestones were transferred to different ages; 67.7% of those transferred were moved to older ages. Approximately 80% of the final milestones had normative data from >1 sources. Social-emotional and cognitive milestones had the least normative data. These criteria and revised checklists can be used to support developmental surveillance, clinical judgment regarding additional developmental screening, and research in developmental surveillance processes. Gaps in developmental data were identified particularly for social-emotional and cognitive milestones." [299]

> *This "wait-and-see" approach causes delays in appropriate evaluation.*

With the revisions, there is now a checklist for every well-child visit from two months to five years of age, with a total of 159 milestones across 12 checklists as compared with the previous 216 milestones across 10 checklists. As summarized by the AAP, the new guidelines reflect the following changes:[300]

- Addition of checklists for ages 15 and 30 months
- Addition of new social and emotional milestones (e.g., "Smiles on their own to get attention" at age four months)
- Removal of vague language such as "may" or "begins" when referring to some milestones
- Removal of duplicate milestones
- Addition of new, open-ended questions for use in discussion with families (e.g., "Is there anything that the child does or does not do that concerns you?")
- Revision and expansion of tips and activities for "developmental promotion and early relational health"

One of the biggest changes to the developmental milestones involves language development, with a number of speech and language milestones pushed up to older age groups. For example, the CDC's 2004 guidelines suggested children should have a 50-word vocabulary, on average, by 24 months of age, but the new guidelines list 30 months as the target age for reaching this milestone. In addition:

- The CDC removed more than half of the milestones from the original 216 milestones (including "tries to use things the right way, like a phone, cup, or book," which was a milestone noted across multiple age groups).
- The CDC added milestone markers to show clearer signs of autism. One example, a social and emotional milestone, is at two months, when babies ordinarily should calm down when spoken to or picked up. Another is at four months, when most babies are smiling on their own to get attention. At 15 months, children should be able to clap when they get excited.
- The CDC moved about one-third of the previous milestones (such as fine motor skills) to older age groups.
- Another change is the removal of crawling as a CDC developmental milestone. This change is controversial because crawling is very important, building up neck strength and control, developing strength for walking, and using both sides of the brain together.

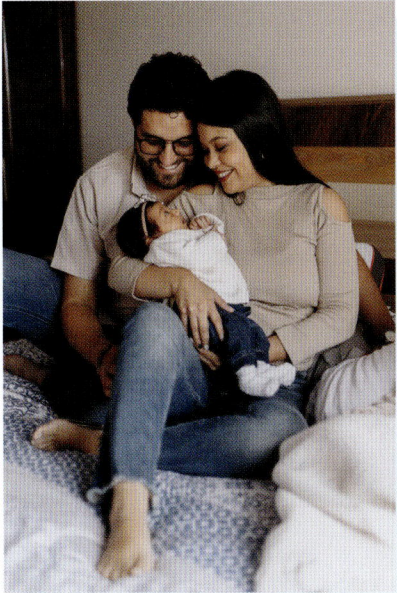
© Fernanda/Adobe Stock

> *The CDC removed more than half of the milestones from the original 216 milestones.*

Although the stated aim of the CDC's revised developmental guidelines is to increase surveillance of potential developmental delays, by moving approximately one-third of the milestones, such as fine motor skills, up to older age groups, the guidelines no longer support early intervention. Closing off opportunities for early assessment, the guidelines may actually worsen children's developmental delays, pushing a child who was originally one standard deviation below the norm to two standard deviations below. By the time someone identifies a problem, the child may need to be caught up even more, which in turn means more time in therapy and increased costs. In short, there are concerns that the guidelines will increase potential setbacks and delay the start of timely interventions.

Early intervention is critical to help families develop strategies to manage behavioral, emotional, social, and educational challenges.[301] Unfortunately, a study published in 2017 in the *Journal of Developmental & Behavioral Pediatrics* found that there were only 1,000 pediatricians in the United States specially trained to treat developmental disorders. The study, involving a national sample of U.S. children's hospitals, identified barriers to evaluation by developmental pediatricians that included long wait times and inadequate Spanish language accommodation. Of the 140 unique programs, only 55% (75 programs) even offered a wait time estimate, which was, on average, nearly five and a half months. Among these, just 62 were able to respond in Spanish within 24 hours of the initial contact, and nearly one-third did not offer any Spanish-language services. A March 2022 phone call to the Children's Hospital of Philadelphia Division of Developmental and Behavioral Pediatrics indicated a wait time of seven months for an initial consultation with a developmental pediatrician. The 2017 study highlighted the need to identify optimal strategies for connecting children displaying developmental concerns with the appropriate evaluation facilities.

> *Early intervention is critical to help families develop strategies to manage behavioral, emotional, social, and educational challenges.*

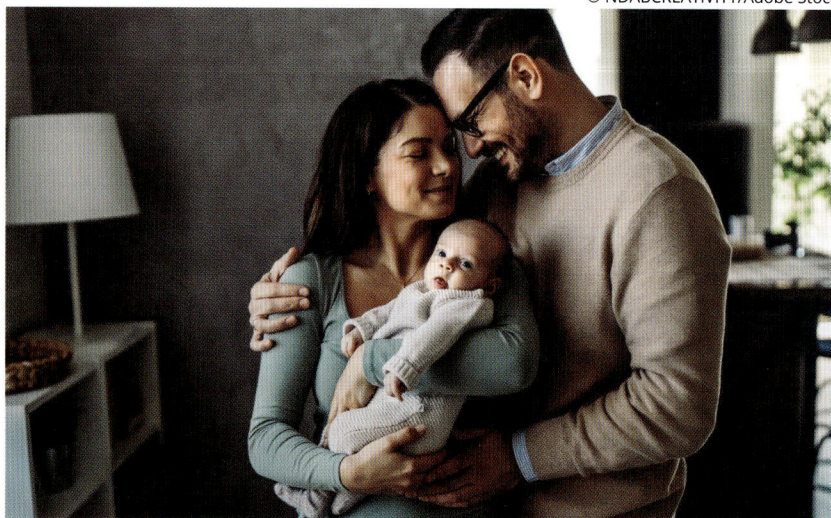

Government researchers who focus on developmental disabilities have noted the pressing need for additional studies to better understand:[302]

- The characteristics of children with developmental disabilities
- The "complex risk factors" associated with such disabilities
- The accessibility of services and interventions "shown to improve long-term outcomes for those diagnosed with a developmental disability"

Unfortunately, there has been no follow-up study even though the measures adopted during SARS-CoV-2—including lockdowns, extensive restrictions to social environments, and facial coverings—appear to have increased the percentage of children with developmental delays.[303] It is essential to honestly investigate the reasons for the increased prevalence of developmental delays and develop better strategies for assessment, intervention, and prevention.

Delays in Language Milestones

One of the most concerning aspects of CDC's revised developmental guidelines is the lowering of standards for speech and language milestones, now pushed to older age groups. It is true

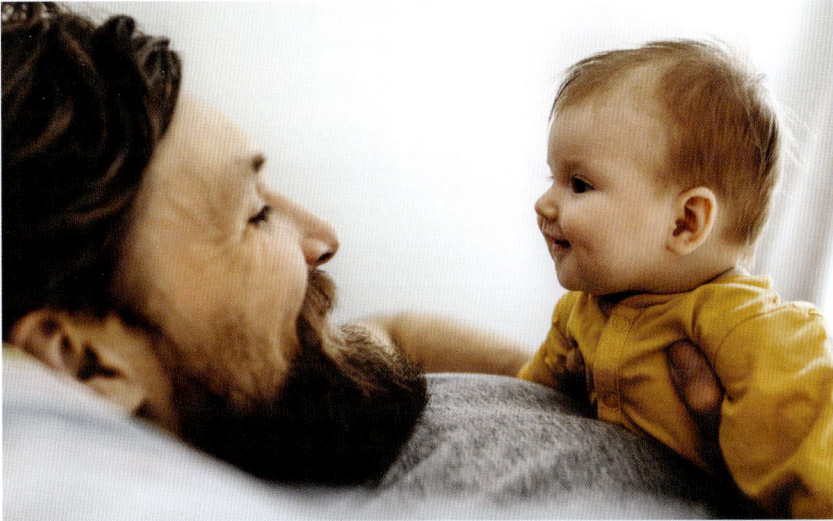

© EVERST/Adobe Stock

that children develop at their own rate, with some children walking and talking earlier and others taking longer, but most children learn skills within a certain age range. A child who takes longer to learn a skill may have a problem. In shifting the milestone of a 50-word vocabulary (on average) from 24 months to 30 months, the CDC guidelines contradict the American Speech-Language-Hearing Association (ASHA), which considers saying less than 50 words at two years old a red flag (see "Signs of Language Problems" on page 94).[304] Lowering the standards for speech and language could prevent a child from getting an Individualized Family Service Plan (IFSP) and could result in a late Individualized Education Plan (IEP) when the child starts school, delaying access to much-needed assessments and services.

> *One of the most concerning aspects of CDC's revised developmental guidelines is the lowering of standards for speech and language milestones, now pushed to older age groups.*

Signs of Language Problems

Language includes speaking, understanding, reading, and writing. A child with a language disorder may have trouble with one or more of the following skills:

- Birth–3 months: Not smiling or playing with others.
- 4–7 months: Not babbling.
- 7–12 months: Making only a few sounds. Not using gestures like waving or pointing.
- 7 months–2 years: Not understanding what others say.
- 12–18 months: Saying only a few words.
- 1½–2 years: Not putting two words together.
- 2 years: Saying fewer than 50 words.
- 2–3 years: Having trouble playing and talking with other children.
- 2½–3 years: Having problems with early reading and writing. For example, your child may not like to draw or look at books.

Source: American Speech-Language-Hearing Association

Children need successful intervention early in life to correct potential language delays and prevent further setbacks. If providers identify a child's developmental delay at 30 months of age, chances are that there will be at least a six-month wait time for intervention, given the current critical shortage of professionals available to properly evaluate the delay.

Speech-language pathologists (SLPs) work with children who have language, speech sound, stuttering, or voice problems. Audiologists help children who have trouble hearing. It is best to find an SLP or audiologist who has earned a Certificate of Clinical Competence (CCC) from ASHA. ASHA-certified SLPs have "CCC-SLP" after their name, and ASHA-certified audiologists have "CCC-A" after their name. The ASHA ProFind website can help parents find an SLP or audiologist.[305]

> *Children need successful intervention early in life to correct potential language delays and prevent further setbacks.*

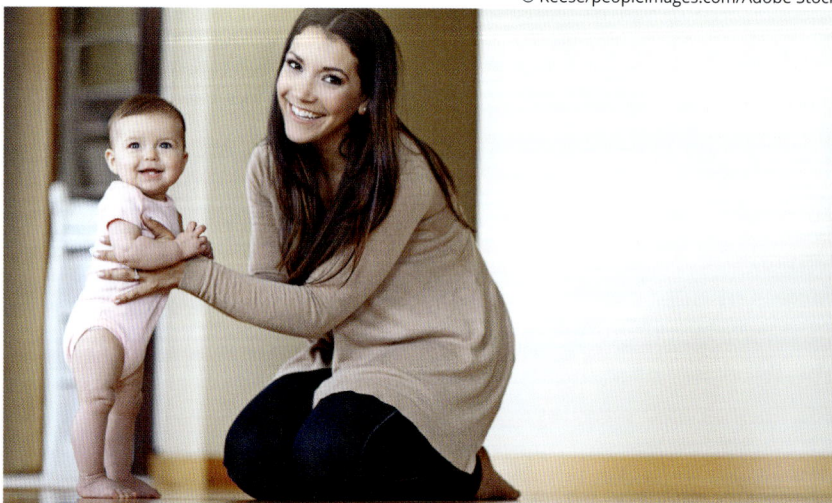

© Reese/peopleimages.com/Adobe Stock

During 2020–2022, many children who suffered from delayed language milestones did not have access to an in-person SLP. Imagine a two-year-old with language delays trying to communicate with a person over a virtual Zoom call, or a child who was able to see a professional, but one or both had to wear a face covering. Sensitivity to facial and vocal emotion is fundamental to children's social competence. Previous research has focused on children's facial emotion recognition, and some studies have investigated non-linguistic vocal emotion processing in childhood.[306] The extent of harm experienced by children during the events of 2020–2022 is incalculable.

Delays in Movement and Gross Motor Milestones

As already mentioned, crawling is an essential milestone, influencing "the motor development that is required for conscious reaching and other movements, the infant's orientation in space and time, multitasking, and cognitive development."[307] A delay in "early unconditioned crawling," says neurosensorimotor expert Svetlana Masgutova, will negatively affect "all other phases of the Crawling Reflex" and may be indicative of a neurodevelopmental concern. Thus, the CDC's removal of crawling from the developmental milestones checklist is both puzzling and counterproductive.

Delays in Cognitive Milestones

Cognitive delays refer to children "whose intellectual function and adaptive behavior are significantly below the expected average for their age."[308] Many factors may contribute to delays in cognitive milestones.

Genetic factors, such as the inheritance of abnormal genes or a chromosomal disorder, are one possible contributor. Examples of chromosomal disorders include Fragile X syndrome, Down syndrome, and phenylketonuria (PKU).

Cognitive delays can also develop as a result of exposures during pregnancy, such as maternal drug or alcohol use. Adverse effects from vaccines administered during pregnancy, such as the flu, Tdap, or COVID shots, also fall into this category. In addition, complications at birth—such as prematurity, a labor complication, or inadequate oxygenation of the infant—can affect cognitive development.

> *The CDC's removal of crawling from the developmental milestones checklist is both puzzling and counterproductive.*

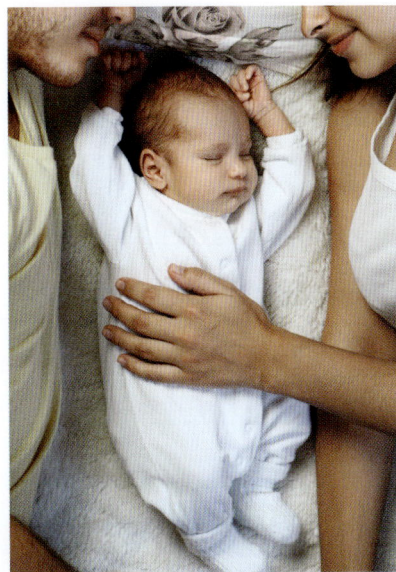

© Artranq/Adobe Stock

95

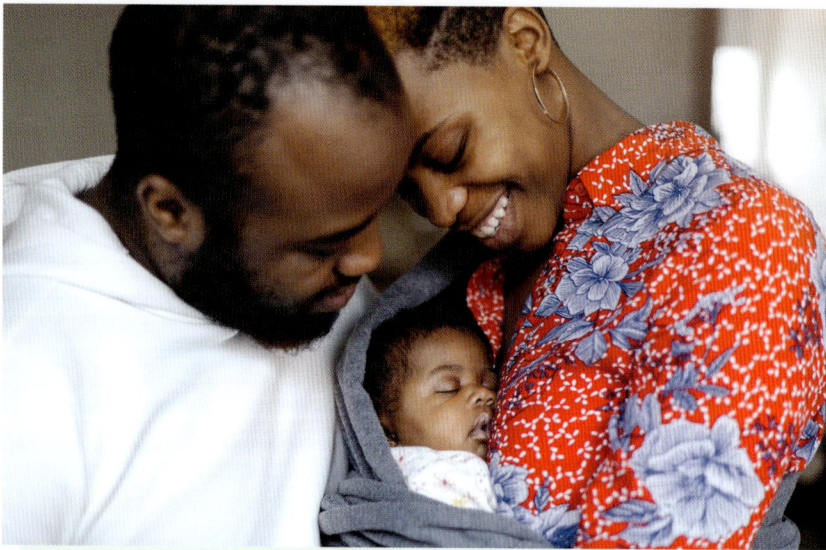

© pikselstock/Adobe Stock

Other contributors to cognitive delays include external factors such as malnutrition and exposure to heavy metals, including in vaccines. A 2010 study found that boys who received thimerosal-containing hepatitis B vaccines as neonates "had threefold greater odds for autism diagnosis compared to boys never vaccinated or vaccinated after the first month of life."[309]

Most often, parents, caregivers, or teachers are the first to identify a concern (see "Signs of Cognitive Developmental Delays"). It is crucial that parents make a primary care physician aware of the concern and request an evaluation of the child, particularly given the limited number of developmental pediatricians in the U.S. and the sometimes lengthy wait times to access their services.

Signs of Cognitive Developmental Delays

Parents can observe some forms of cognitive delay as early as 24 months of age:

- Sitting, crawling, or walking later than other children
- Having difficulty speaking
- Having a short attention span
- Being unable to remember things
- Displaying a lack of curiosity
- Having trouble understanding social rules or the consequences of behavior
- Having trouble thinking logically
- Exhibiting infantile behavior that persists into the preschool and school years
- Lacking age-appropriate adaptive or self-help skills

Source: "What Are Cognitive Developmental Delays," The Warren Center, accessed Jan. 5, 2023, thewarrencenter.org/help-information/cognitive/what-are-cognitive-developmental-delays.

Other contributors to cognitive delays include external factors such as malnutrition and exposure to heavy metals, including in vaccines.

Developmental pediatricians evaluate and diagnose cognitive delays or disorders by assessing both intellectual functioning (using sensitive tests that measure a child's ability to learn, solve problems, and understand the world) and adaptive functioning (the ability to develop independent living skills). Following a thorough evaluation, a child may qualify for early intervention services. The most beneficial strategy is to use an individualized multidisciplinary team approach that encompasses intervention, family therapy, and therapies for the child—which may include occupational, nutrition, speech, and/or physical therapy. The goal is to support the child and family to achieve goals that are realistic and emphasize health and happiness.

Vaccine Ingredients as Environmental Toxins

A 2015 article in the *Annual Review of Public Health* explains why various environmental toxins pose such a threat to the developing brain:

"The developing brain is particularly vulnerable to environmental toxins. The blood–brain of the developing brain is not fully formed, and it is more permeable to toxins than is the mature brain. The rapid growth of the brain during the second trimester of fetal development is followed by neuronal migration, differentiation, proliferation, and pruning throughout early childhood. Growing cells are more vulnerable to toxins, and the brain forms over a longer period than do other organs. Finally, the brain is composed of many different types of neurons, each type having a distinct growth phase and potentially a different toxicity profile." [310]

> " *The goal is to support the child and family to achieve goals that are realistic and emphasize health and happiness.* "

© Looker_Studio/Adobe Stock

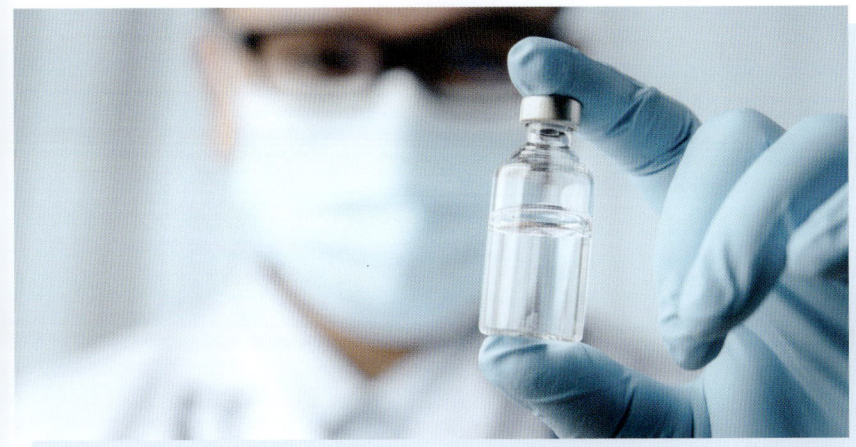

The alarming statistics on the prevalence of developmental delays and their increase raise many questions about which environmental toxins might be contributors. The surge in developmental delays—and in many other chronic illnesses that plague today's children—began in the early 1990s and coincides notably with the ballooning of the childhood vaccination schedule. In the 1970s and 1980s, American children typically received three types of vaccines against seven diseases,[311] but by 2017, they were receiving (beginning prenatally and continuing on the day of birth and up to age 18) up to 56 doses of injected or oral vaccines for 16 diseases.[312] Moreover, whereas only about half of American two-year-olds completed their recommended series of vaccines in the late 1980s,[313] by 2017, about nine in ten children under three were receiving all or most recommended vaccines.[314]

Bypassing the body's normal defenses, vaccines introduce into the body a range of toxic and potentially troublesome ingredients—including disclosed substances as well as undisclosed ingredients and contaminants.[315] A partial list of vaccine components includes:

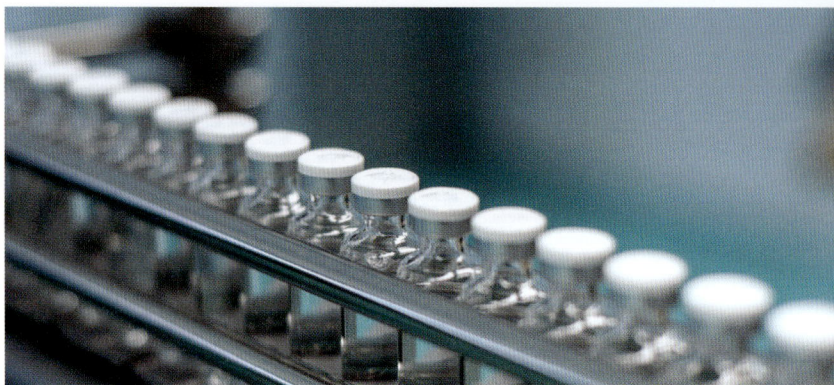

© Konstantin Chimbai/Adobe Stock

- Neurotoxic metals such as aluminum and mercury
- Carcinogenic formaldehyde
- Gene DNA fragments
- Carrier proteins
- Glyphosate
- Antibiotics such as neomycin
- Squalene nanoemulsions
- Metallic micro- and nanoparticles
- With the advent of Covid injections, lipid nanoparticles that encapsulate messenger RNA (mRNA) and are coated with polyethylene glycol (PEG)[316,317,318,319,320,321,322,323,324,325]

When combined, these ingredients likely have synergistic effects that could result in exponentially greater adverse effects on the brain.[326,327]

Unfortunately, analyses of the Covid injections suggest that dubious ingredients and "lousy" manufacturing processes are par for the course and that at least some vaccines are "toxic by design."[328]

> *Bypassing the body's normal defenses, vaccines introduce into the body a range of toxic and potentially troublesome ingredients.*

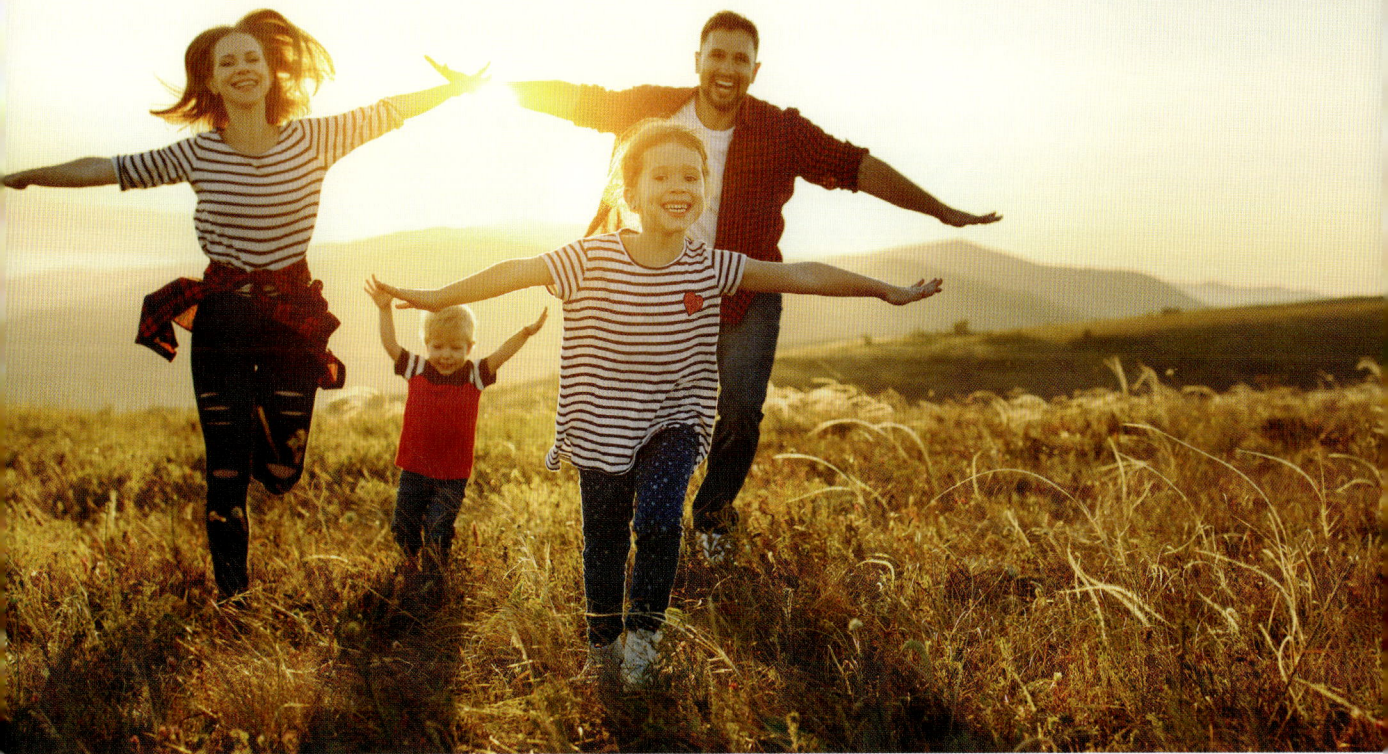

Chapter Seven: Environmental Exposures

"[E]vidence has accumulated over the past century that implicates ubiquitous, low-level exposures to an ever-growing litany of environmental toxins in the development of diminished birth weight, shortened gestation, intellectual deficits, and mental disorders in children." — **Bruce P. Lanphear, MD, MPH**

In recent years, people's awareness has increased regarding the negative health effects of environmental toxins ranging from synthetic chemicals, neurotoxic metals, and fluoride to electromagnetic fields (EMFs).

Although exposure to environmental toxins can pose a health threat to everyone, the effects are particularly detrimental to developing fetuses and young children. Many of these exposures take place unknowingly within the home.

It is important for parents to understand where exposures most often occur and what they can do to protect themselves and their children.

In this chapter, we will:

- Review some common environmental toxins
- Discuss where they are found
- Describe how they impact health
- Outline basic steps parents can take to mitigate exposures for both themselves and their children

> *Many of these exposures take place unknowingly within the home.*

Synthetic Chemicals

Synthetic chemicals are present in many everyday products, such as plastics, mattresses, carpets, cookware, and food.[329] Many of these chemicals have a broad impact on health and may disrupt hormones, damage vital organs, and even cause cancer. Some of the more common chemicals known to be dangerous to humans are phthalates, flame retardants, bisphenol A (BPA), and polyfluoroalkyl substances (PFAS).

Phthalates

Manufacturers use a group of chemicals called phthalates in many plastic products as well as some cosmetics,[330] including vinyl flooring, shower curtains, plastic packaging, wood finishes, detergents, soaps, and shampoos. Exposure to phthalates can disrupt the endocrine system by mimicking or blocking male and female sex hormones.

Pregnant women and young children are particularly vulnerable to phthalate exposure because the chemicals can cross the placenta and interfere with development at crucial stages. Phthalates most commonly enter the body through ingestion or inhalation. Young children spend a lot of time on the floor and often put objects in their mouths to explore, which can place them at greater risk of exposure.

Parents can reduce their child's phthalate exposure by checking labels and purchasing products that are phthalate-free, as well as being cognizant of what items the child is putting into their mouth. Additionally, parents can use a vacuum with a HEPA filter or a wet mop to regularly clean floors and floor dust, which may accumulate phthalates as phthalate-containing products degrade.

> *Many of these chemicals have a broad impact on health and may disrupt hormones, damage vital organs, and even cause cancer.*

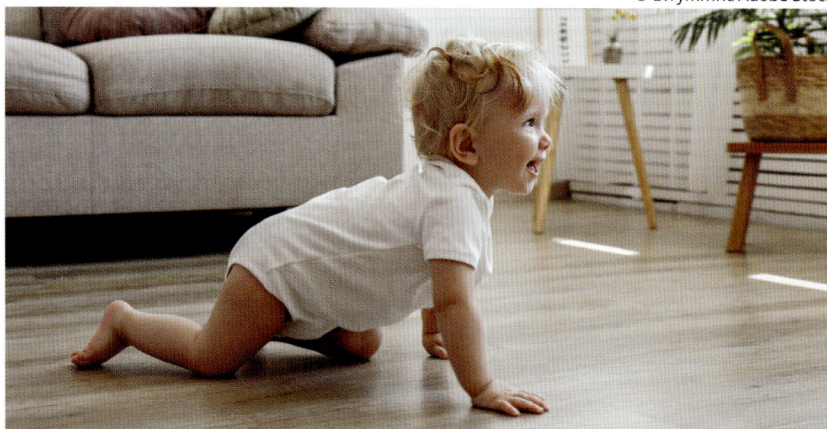

© Evrymmnt/Adobe Stock

Flame Retardants

Consumers commonly encounter flame retardants, a group of chemicals intended to reduce burning in the event of a fire, in furniture (such as couches and mattresses), curtains, electronic devices, and construction materials.[331] Flame retardants disrupt immune function, cause endocrine dysfunction, and can be associated with cancer.

Fetuses and children in early stages of development are most vulnerable to the effects of these toxic chemicals. Over time, products that contain flame retardants break down and turn into dust, at which point children may inhale or ingest them. Similarly to phthalates, parents can reduce their own and their children's exposure to flame retardants by purchasing products that are flame-retardant-free. Today, safe mattresses, car seats, and furniture are available from select manufacturers. As a child gets older, parents should be sure to continue reading product descriptions and labels to find items that reduce the child's exposure to flame retardants.

Bisphenol A (BPA)

Manufacturers use BPA in the manufacture of plastics, with BPA-containing products including some canned food linings, shopping receipts, water bottles, food containers, and children's toys.[332] Most of the time, BPA enters the body when someone consumes food that has been in contact with BPA-coated surfaces or places BPA-containing objects in the mouth. A pregnant mother exposed to BPA can also expose her developing fetus. BPA is another chemical that interferes with hormones, namely estrogen. BPA mimics estrogen by binding to estrogen receptors on the surface of cells.

In babies and young children, BPA can affect brain development, thyroid function, and behavior. Steps that parents can take to lessen their children's BPA exposure include avoiding canned foods, not heating plastic food containers or baby bottles, and purchasing wood rather than plastic toys.

Unfortunately, parents also need to beware of products labeled "BPA-free," as manufacturers often replace BPA with even more toxic chemicals in the same chemical family.

> *In babies and young children, BPA can affect brain development, thyroid function, and behavior.*

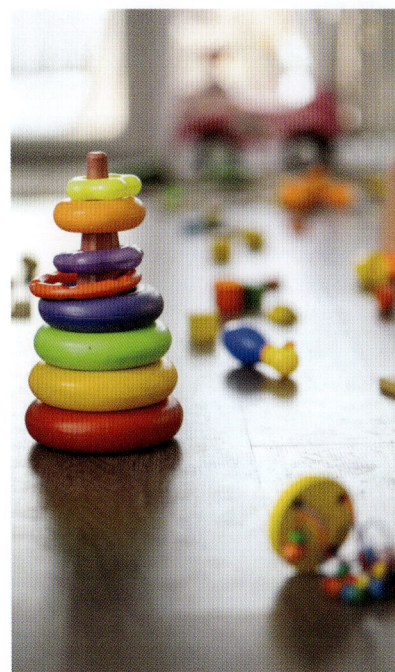

© Evgenia Tiplyashina/Adobe Stock

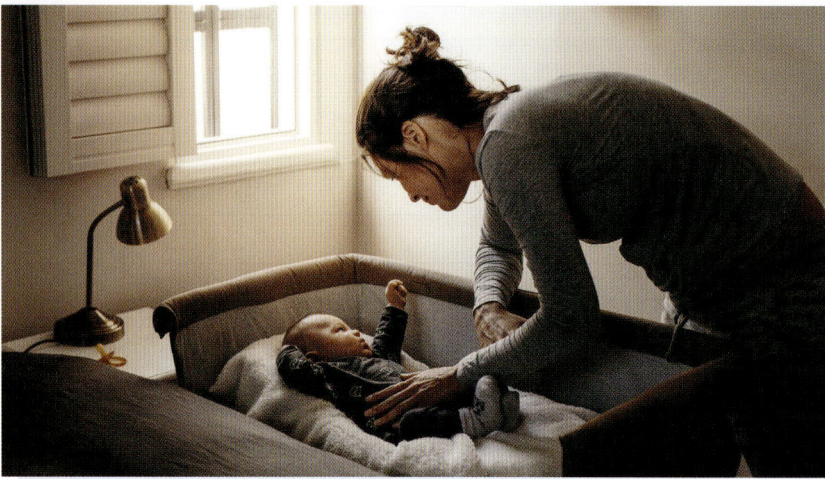

© Jacob Lund/Adobe Stock

Polyfluoroalkyl Substances (PFAS)

PFAS are a group of chemicals that are pervasive in the environment,[333] sometimes referred to as "forever chemicals" due to their ability to persist for years without breaking down. Manufacturers use PFAS in non-stick cookware, clothes, carpets, foams, and construction and electronic products. Due to their widespread use, PFAS have contaminated water supplies, soil, and the air.

Testing in late 2022 identified detectable levels of PFAS chemicals in almost a third of tested baby products.[334] Products tested included baby bedding, bibs, diaper changing pads, and snack bags.

PFAS chemicals accumulate in the body and are associated with decreased immune function, cancer, low birth weight, birth defects, and high blood pressure and pre-eclampsia in pregnant women. Parents can lessen PFAS exposure by avoiding products coated with PFAS, such as non-stick cookware, waterproof clothing, and stain-resistant carpets. It is also important to check the quality of the household water supply to ensure no PFAS contamination.

Neurotoxic Metals

Among the metals of concern to fetuses and young children are lead, arsenic, mercury, and aluminum.[335]

> " Due to their widespread use, PFAS have contaminated water supplies, soil, and the air. "

Lead

Manufacturers used lead for decades to make products ranging from paint to gasoline.[336] During the 1970s, as lead's detrimental effects came to greater public awareness, companies and legislators began taking steps to eliminate it from many products. Notwithstanding considerable progress in reducing lead exposure, lead is still widely present and continues to pose a health risk for many. Exposure to lead, particularly in young children, can lead to decreased intelligence, behavioral problems, stunted growth, abdominal pain, attention problems, and delayed speech. The Environmental Protection Agency (EPA) also notes that some lead compounds are likely carcinogens and observes that in adults, even "[s]mall amounts of lead cause hypertension … and permanent mental dysfunction."[337]

Sources of lead today include old house paint (the government banned lead-based paints for residential use in 1978), contaminated drinking water, ceramic pottery, and old toys. Lead has been detected in some baby foods and candy.[338] In addition, manufacturers use lead in the flexible coatings of electrical wires and cables. (Additional materials of concern used in the wire and cable industry include other metals such as cadmium and antimony, brominated flame retardants, and phthalates.[339]) The EPA explains, "Lead-based heat stabilizers are added to PVC for wire and cable applications because they provide long-term thermal stability and electrical resistance with low water absorption."[340] The agency admits that these stabilizers "have potential adverse health and environmental effects due to the known toxicity of lead."

> *Lead has been detected in some baby foods and candy.*

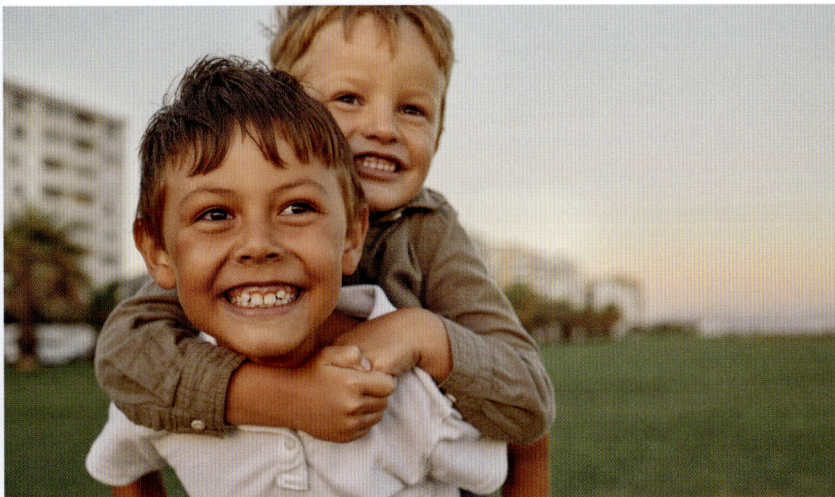

It is important to know whether one's home contains lead-based paint and, if it does, take measures to protect children from exposure. Other protection measures that parents can take include checking local water quality reports (or having well water tested), making homemade baby food, and becoming very cognizant of the items a child is placing in their mouth. Stringing Christmas tree lights is often a family activity, but because many of the wires are coated in lead, some medical websites advise that only parents handle them—"ideally while wearing gloves"—and keep them away from young children.[341]

Arsenic

Arsenic can accumulate naturally in soil and water or it can be a result of industrial processes such as mining.[342] Today, the most common exposures to arsenic are through drinking water and through foods cultivated in soil containing arsenic. Arsenic-based compounds were in common use in both industry and agriculture throughout the 20th century, and some researchers have expressed concern regarding potential "delayed effects" of exposure.[343]

Arsenic is a known carcinogen, and exposure is also associated with cardiovascular illness, diabetes, and developmental problems. Parents can protect children from arsenic exposure by making sure their drinking water is free from contamination and by limiting foods known to contain elevated levels of arsenic, such as rice.

Mercury

Mercury is a highly toxic metal that occurs both naturally and with industrial manufacturing, resulting in widespread pollution in the environment.[344] Today, some of the main sources of mercury include electrical products, old thermometers, amalgam dental fillings, fluorescent light bulbs, and seafood products.

> *Arsenic is a known carcinogen, and exposure is also associated with cardiovascular illness, diabetes, and developmental problems.*

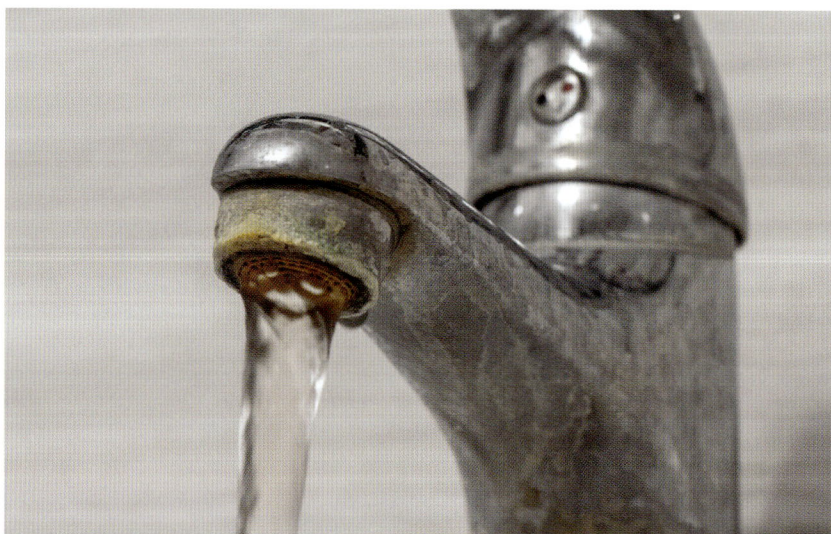

© Serhii/Adobe Stock

According to the FDA, the mercury preservative thimerosal (which is 49% mercury) is still present in varying amounts in some childhood vaccines.[345] For example, inactivated influenza vaccines that come in multidose vials contain 24.5 to 25 micrograms of mercury per full dose; the CDC recommends two such flu shots for children at six and seven months of age and "does not preferentially recommend vaccines that do not contain thimerosal."[346] Moreover, the FDA states that babies are more likely than not to get thimerosal-containing flu shots because "the amount of thimerosal-preservative-free [influenza] vaccine that is available based on current manufacturing capacity is well below the number of doses needed to fully vaccinate this age group."[347] Meanwhile, other "thimerosal-reduced" childhood vaccines use thimerosal in the manufacturing process, leaving what the FDA refers to as "trace amounts" (defined as up to one microgram of mercury per dose). Because of mercury's known neurotoxicity, scientists have argued that "[f]rom a toxicological point of view, the Intentional exposure of humans ... to any form of mercury is illogical."[348]

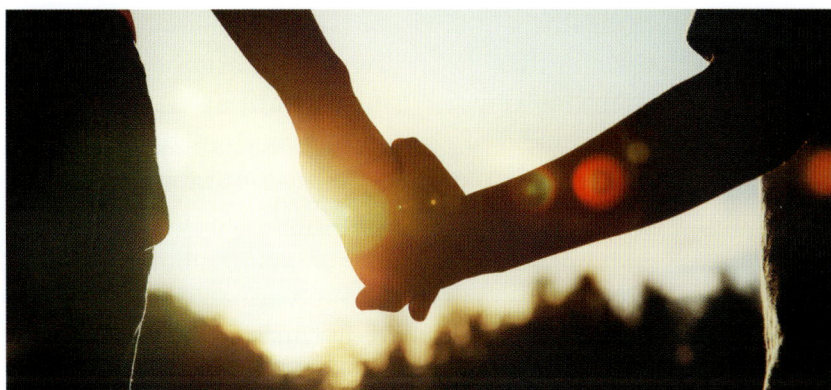

© nadezhdal906/Adobe Stock

Children are extremely vulnerable to mercury exposure in utero, through breast milk, or through vaccination. These and other avenues of mercury exposure can result in learning deficits, lower IQ, organ damage, vision and hearing problems, epilepsy, autism spectrum disorders, and more.[349]

In addition to evaluating the mercury risks of childhood vaccines, parents may wish to avoid use of fluorescent light bulbs, including compact fluorescent light bulbs (CFLs), which contain mercury. Breaking a bulb of this type releases dangerous mercury vapor; the EPA cautions that vacuuming debris from a broken fluorescent bulb "could spread mercury-containing powder or mercury vapor."[350] Do not throw away broken or used-up CFLs in household trash, as the mercury they contain can taint local water supplies; they must be taken to designated retailers or hazardous waste recycling locations.

> " Children are extremely vulnerable to mercury exposure in utero, through breast milk, or through vaccination. "

The same public health authorities that claim that thimerosal-containing baby shots are safe recommend that mothers limit their intake of mercury-containing seafood while pregnant or breastfeeding. They also advise that children under age 12 not consume more than 8 to 12 ounces of higher-mercury-level seafood (for example, tuna and swordfish) per week. Fish that are low in mercury include sardines, salmon, and cod.

Aluminum

The modern world—what aluminum expert Dr. Christopher Exley refers to as the "aluminum age"—contains many routes of aluminum exposure, including through food and cookware but also "via the skin" (for example, in antiperspirants) "or the nose or the lung"[351]—as well as through vaccination. Across many studies, Exley has demonstrated aluminum's "incontrovertible" neurotoxicity, additionally describing aluminum as an excitotoxin (a substance that overstimulates the brain) and a mutagen (something that causes genetic mutations).[352]

For babies and young children, vaccination constitutes a significant exposure. About 80% of vaccines rely on one or more aluminum adjuvants (aluminum compounds added to vaccines to augment their immune impact).[353] A 2015 study conducted by CDC and Kaiser Permanente showed that for fully vaccinated two-year-olds born after 2004, exposure to aluminum was 11% to 26% higher than for children "under-vaccinated" before age two.[354] This has resulted in a high degree of chronic aluminum toxicity. Dr. Exley has stated, "Exposure to aluminum through a vaccine is, in comparison to diet, an acute exposure."[355]

Fluoride

The U.S. is one of only 11 countries in the world where more than half of the population consumes artificially fluoridated drinking water, and more people in the U.S. drink fluoridated water "than the rest of the world combined."[356] Fourteen other countries have smaller-scale water fluoridation programs.

About 80% of vaccines rely on one or more aluminum adjuvants.

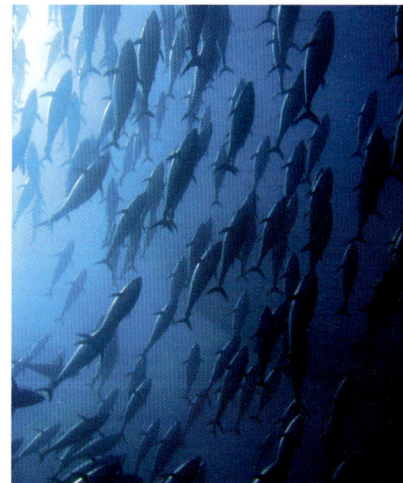

© Guido/Adobe Stock

A preponderance of evidence indicates that in utero and postpartum fluoride exposure lowers IQ and produces neurodevelopmental toxicity "comparable to the effects of lead."[357] A 2019 study showed that when mothers were exposed during pregnancy to what the CDC defines as "optimally fluoridated water," it led to lower IQ scores in their offspring.[358] The researchers noted that fluoride can cross the placenta, accumulate in brain regions involved in learning and memory, and alter brain proteins and neurotransmitters.

In addition to effects on cognition, studies link fluoride to preterm birth,[359] behavioral symptoms of inattention,[360] and health risks such as bone disease and bone cancer.[361,362]

The "one dose fits all" approach to water fluoridation poses particular risks to children. The International Academy of Oral Medicine and Toxicology (IAOMT) states:

"This blanket approach fails to address the smaller size of infants and children and the larger proportions of water and other fluoridated beverages they drink. Significantly, a formula-fed infant drinks its weight in water every three to four days, resulting in the most vulnerable members of the population consuming by far the largest dose of fluoride." [363]

Notably, water fluoridation also increases the toxicity of dietary aluminum exposures. In fact, Exley describes aluminum as the "elephant in the room" where water fluoridation is concerned, observing that "Fluoride increases the absorption of aluminum across the human gut and hence increases the body burden of aluminum."[364]

> *A preponderance of evidence indicates that in utero and postpartum fluoride exposure lowers IQ.*

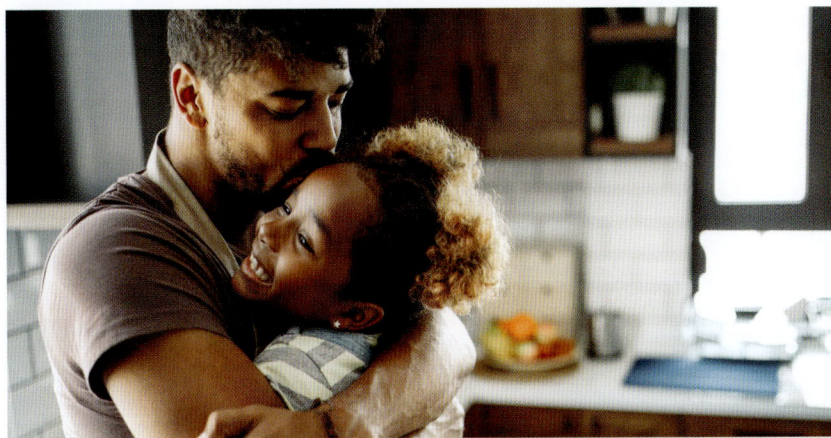

Electromagnetic Fields (EMFs)

A wide variety of home electronic products emit EMFs,[365] a type of non-ionizing radiation that is invisible to the naked eye and undetectable unless using special equipment to measure levels. Common sources of EMFs include power lines, Wi-Fi, cell phones, wireless tablets, cell phone towers, so-called "smart meters," and other wireless devices. For example, the multiple antennas in wireless tablets—popular with young children—emit constant bursts of pulsed radiation (up to 900 times per hour), even when not in use.[366]

Historically, this constant EMF exposure is a relatively recent phenomenon. Even so, there are thousands of studies linking EMFs to significant adverse biological effects, including evidence that associates EMF exposure with cancer.[367]

According to the National Cancer Institute, three factors increase children's cell phone risks in comparison to those of adults:[368]

- Children's nervous systems "are still developing and, therefore, [are] more vulnerable to factors that may cause cancer."

- Children have smaller heads "and consequently have a greater proportional exposure to the field of radiofrequency radiation that is emitted by cell phones."

- Children have "the potential of accumulating more years of cell phone exposure than adults do."

Parents can take steps to limit their children's EMF exposure, for example, by using hardwired Internet connections in the home instead of Wi-Fi, and not allowing children to play with parents' cell phones or tablets, including iPads. Make sure children never have a cell phone near their body, and avoid taking children into places that are in close proximity to cell towers and high-voltage power lines. Parents who do use Wi-Fi in the home should turn it off when not in use, and particularly at night during sleep. For multiple reasons, many health experts also warn against using microwave ovens.[369]

For more information on these exposures and their impacts on children's health, see the free Children's Health Defense eBook, *The Sickest Generation: The Facts Behind the Children's Health Crisis and Why It Needs to End* (second edition), available at the Children's Health Defense website.[370]

> *There are thousands of studies linking EMFs to significant adverse biological effects, including evidence that associates EMF exposure with cancer.*

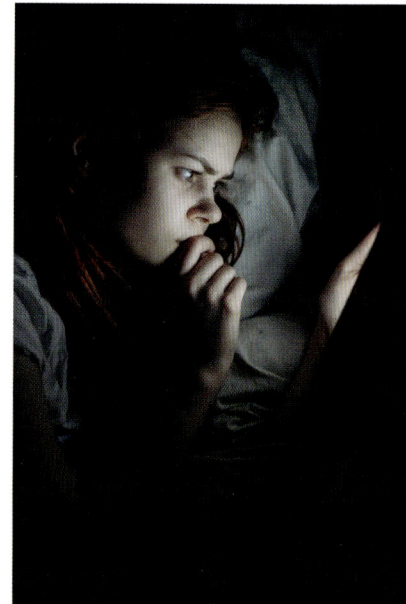

© SHOTPRIME STUDIO/Adobe Stock

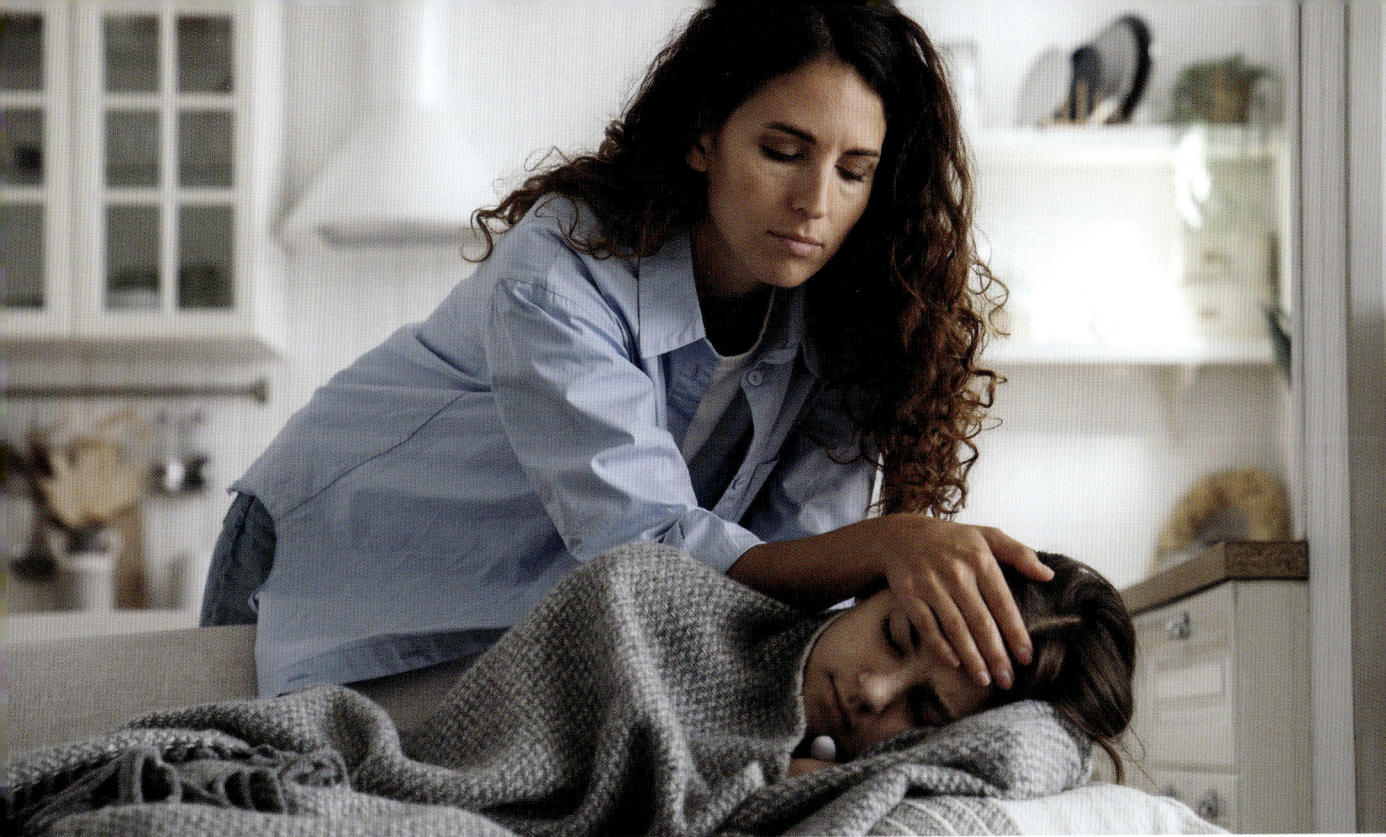

Chapter Eight: Childhood Illness

"Too often, the risk of careless or needless medical intervention is greater than the dangers of the illness itself." — **Dr. Robert S. Mendelsohn**

Most acute illness is beneficial in the sense that it allows people, and especially children, to undergo repair and restoration. Parents often observe that after an illness, a child goes through a developmental level change and experiences a refreshing sense of vitality. What this means is that parents generally need not be fearful when their child feels sick. As Hippocrates said, "Nature itself is the best physician." At the same time, parents know their child best; if an illness appears serious or life-threatening, they should seek professional medical help as soon as possible.

In this chapter, we will:

- Describe the important role of fever

- Review ways that parents can provide comfort and support during a child's illness

- Describe considerations regarding the use of over-the-counter and prescription drugs

- Discuss warning signs that may call for medical attention

> *Parents generally need not be fearful when their child feels sick.*

Detoxification and Restoration

A child's immune system is constantly operating and restoring itself. Inflammation is a natural process that destroys and removes toxins and waste from the body through coughing, sneezing, vomiting, fever, diarrhea, and the buildup of mucus. When inflammation arises, sometimes accompanied by a fever, it is an opportunity for cleansing and healing.

A fever helps the body by filtering out toxins and necessitating rest, offering an opportunity to strengthen the immune system. A fever stimulates immunological resistance, thermoregulation, and blood circulation, and is a healthy response to the presence of toxicity in the body. Dr. Aviva Romm describes fever as "part of a natural and healthy inflammatory response that mobilizes white blood cells, antibodies, and cytokines to fight infection."[371]

With fevers, the golden rule is to not fight the temperature but "treat the whole child." Actions taken to lower a fever and inhibit undesired symptoms deprive the body of an important mechanism of overcoming the illness.[372] Rushing children into getting better can be counterproductive, causing them to suffer repeated bouts of the same illness.

When a fever is present, parents can dress their child warmly with layers of either cotton or wool.[373] For higher fevers (103 degrees Fahrenheit or higher), most doctors will push fever reducers (antipyretics); however, growing controversy surrounds the pediatric use of acetaminophen-containing antipyretics like Tylenol,[374] with some studies also linking maternal use during pregnancy to autism or other problems in offspring.[375] Applying a cool washcloth to the forehead is a way to provide relief. Herbs that are safe for babies and helpful for fever—in teas or tinctures—include chamomile, catnip, lemon balm, ginger root, spearmint, and elder blossom (see Dr. Romm's discussion of how to use these herbs at her website).[376] The Weston A. Price Foundation offers other suggestions as well.

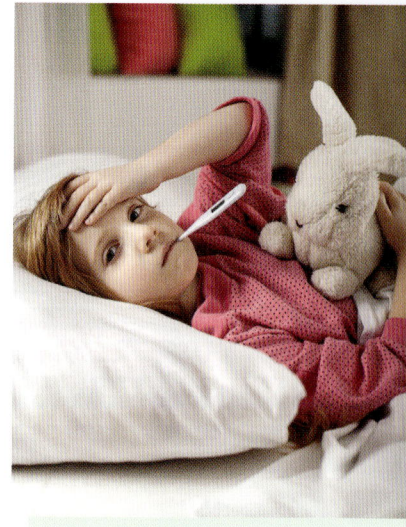

© V&P Photo Studio/Adobe Stock

> *Actions taken to lower a fever and inhibit undesired symptoms deprive the body of an important mechanism of overcoming the illness.*

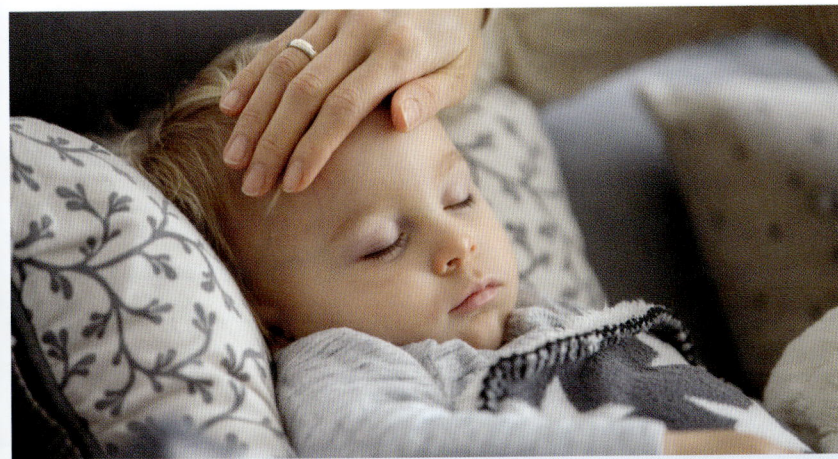

© Tomsickova/Adobe Stock

Hydration is particularly crucial during a fever.

When ill, it is important for children to get plenty of water and sleep,[377,378] which help the body fight off illness. Children should drink as much as they desire during this time. Hydration is particularly crucial during a fever. Hot drinks such as tea with honey and lemon can be helpful. Warm soups and bone broths are also supportive to a body undergoing the healing process. In addition to nutritional and herbal approaches, homeopathy can be a helpful and nontoxic way to support children during illness.

When parents support their child's immune system through love and care instead of fear, it can be a breeze for the child to heal from illness. Surrounding a sick child with love and attention can support physical healing as well as emotional well-being.

Touch from loved ones provides comfort and connection when a child is experiencing suppressed vitality. One long-time family physician has stated,

"[T]he most important thing I have observed in determining the outcome of a child's illness is the attitude of the parents. If the parents have a deep belief that their child is strong and that the illness, if it doesn't become too severe, will serve the child in his future development, their attitude of resolve and confidence will translate into an environment of peacefulness and effectiveness that truly allows the child to rest and to comfortably go through the process." [379]

Medications and Warning Signs

Most of the time, according to former family practice physician Dr. Philip Incao, parents should hesitate before using medications such as antibiotics, aspirin, or ibuprofen, because they suppress symptoms and potentially prolong the illness.[380] When doctors prescribe antibiotics for illnesses such as ear infections, for example, they rarely tell parents about the counterproductive longer-term consequences, which—according to gut specialist Dr. Natasha Campbell-McBride—include destroying beneficial gut bacteria and laying the groundwork "for the next [ear infection] to come."[381] For ear infections, Campbell-McBride recommends that parents stick with tried-and-true home remedies such as dressing the child warmly and keeping them indoors until the ear infection resolves, providing hot drinks (either water with lemon and honey or herbal teas such as chamomile), using garlic-olive oil drops (parents can make these at home or purchase them at natural food stores), or "the old onion remedy" (a chopped onion wrapped in cotton cloth, warmed, and placed on the child's ear).

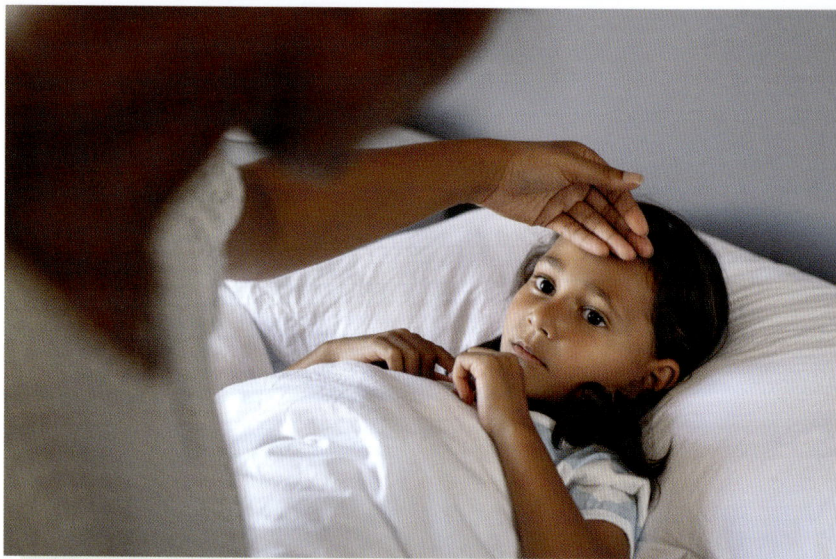

© Rido/Adobe Stock

Dr. Aviva Jill Romm's 2003 book, *Naturally Healthy Babies and Children: A Commonsense Guide to Herbal Remedies, Nutrition, and Health* recommends medical intervention under the following circumstances:

"If a child is severely ill, hemorrhaging, unconscious or displaying symptoms of a serious illness the parents should seek immediate medical care. If a child is not responding to the treatment of a mild condition, and the condition persists or worsens, medical care may be required. Some conditions such as meningitis, appendicitis, bacterial pneumonia, and blood infections can progress rapidly. Symptoms to watch out for include fever, stiff neck, severe abdominal pain, red streaks emanating from a wound and an unremitting fever and/or cough accompanied by severe chest pain." [382]

> *Most of the time... parents should hesitate before using medications such as antibiotics, aspirin, or ibuprofen, because they suppress symptoms and potentially prolong the illness.*

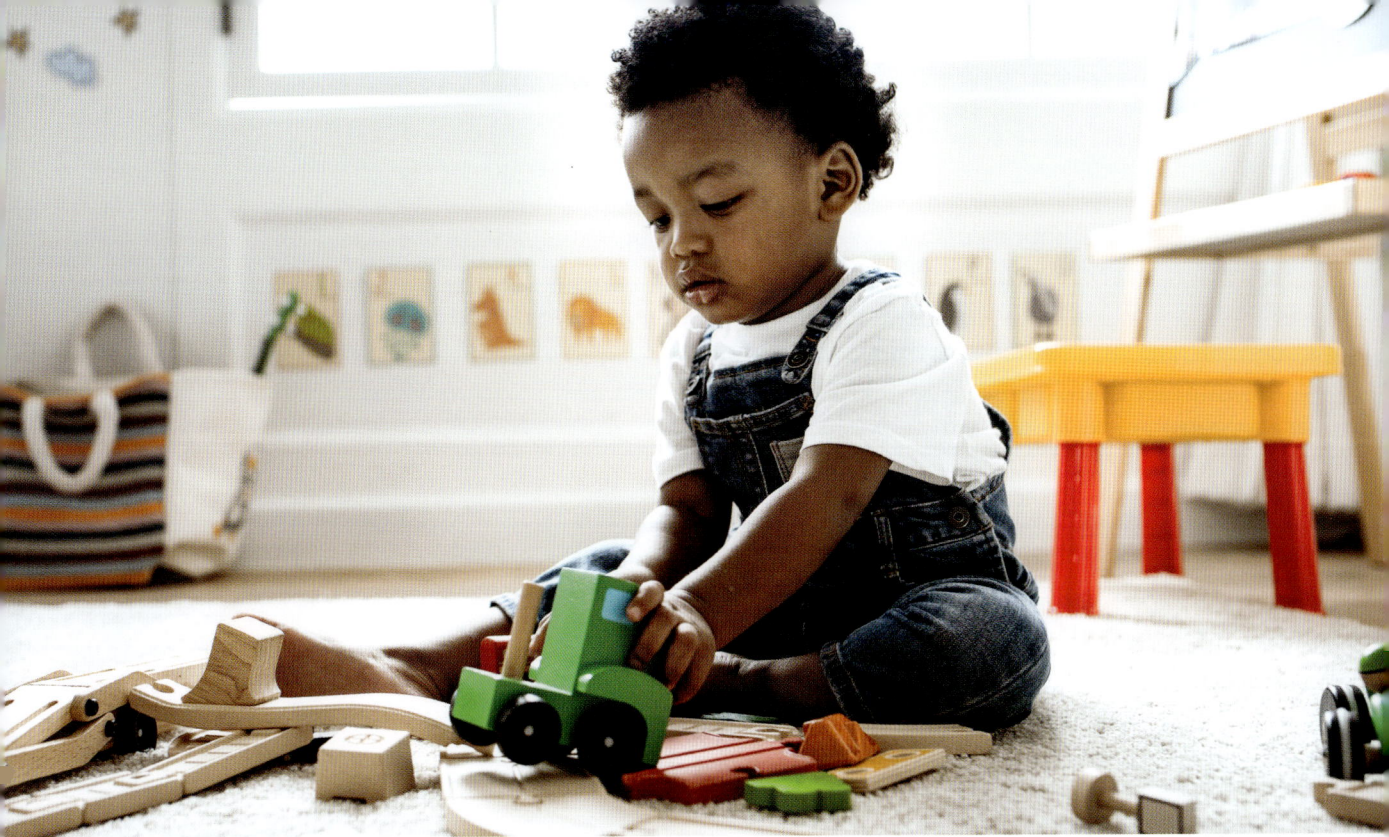

Chapter Nine: Toys

"Play is a child's work." — **Alfred Adler**

Playing with toys represents an enjoyable activity for children, but in addition, toys are learning tools which can help children develop problem-solving and motor skills. Toys also foster a child's intuitive and creative development.

The National Association for the Education of Young Children (NAEYC) recommends keeping in mind a child's stage of development and abilities and choosing toys that are age-appropriate.[383]

However, every child is on their own developmental path, and they do not always conform to what is expected of them for their age group.

In this chapter, we will:

- Explain the importance of imaginative play
- Describe the types of play and toys appropriate during the first few years
- Review toys and toy materials that can be harmful to children's health
- Suggest types of toys that are not harmful

> " *Toys also foster a child's intuitive and creative development.* "

The Importance of Imaginative Play

Stimulating the imagination is one of the backbones of learning. Over time, imaginative play will cultivate concentration, support language development, and offer an energized approach to problem-solving.

If adults force a child to conform to intellectual pursuits and standards before the child has developed their capacity for creativity, imagination, and fantasy, it may inhibit the child's love of learning.

The First Few Years

From birth to six months of age, children find imagery and facial expressions captivating. At this stage of development, parents can enjoy being facially expressive when talking and singing to their baby.

Infants are also interested in objects that they can hold, suck on, and shake. Rattles, squeeze toys, and teething toys are appropriate for this stage of development.

From seven months to one year of age, children like to explore and roll over, scoot, bounce, and stand. At this stage, they can understand their name and concepts such as "playing pretend." Baby dolls, puppets, and wooden vehicles with wheels are appropriate toys for this age group, as well as large soft blocks and wooden cubes, which allow children to build and construct according to their imagination.

A one-year-old child also loves to experiment and enjoys stories and playing with other children.

A distinctive stage in development occurs when a child turns two. Two-year-olds become better able to communicate, have more control of their hands and fingers, and have a heightened interest in jumping, climbing, and tumbling.

By age three, some children may be preschoolers. At this point, they enjoy talking and asking questions. They are curious about their environment, and they like to play and share with other children.

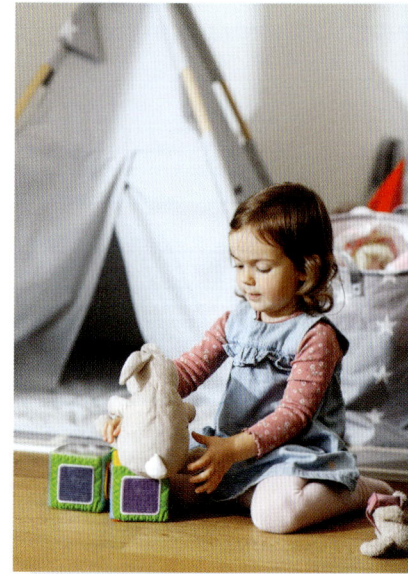

> **A one-year-old child also loves to experiment and enjoys stories and playing with other children.**

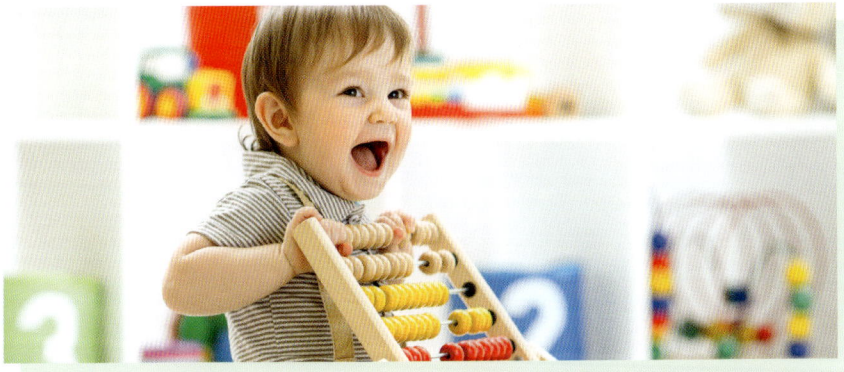

© Oksana Kuzmina/Adobe Stock

Toys to Avoid

Numerous materials involved in the production of toys can be harmful to children's health. It is best to shy away from toys containing plastic. Toys made from plastic likely contain phthalates or BPA; research has linked both to cancer, hormone disruption, and developmental problems.[384]

The National Center for Healthy Housing recommends that families also shy away from painted toys, which may contain lead and other heavy metals linked to developmental impairments.[385]

Parents may also wish to avoid toys incorporating themes that normalize violence or inhibit the imagination.

Better Options

Parents may ask, "What toys can I buy that are not harmful to my baby?"

One safe option are wooden toys produced from ethically sourced forests that are free of plastic, batteries, and lead paint, available at sustainable toy shops. From wooden puzzles and rattles to blocks, dollhouses, and slides, there are numerous options for appropriate toys for each stage of development with simple and unadorned designs to effectively foster a child's imagination. Toys made from safe recycled materials or bamboo are also great choices.

Materials such as beeswax and silk are great creative instruments that foster children's creative development and capture their imagination.

Parents also can make their own toys. Allowing children to participate in cooking, gardening, and other activities that give children an opportunity to explore the world through experience is another way for them to play creatively while developing self-confidence.

> *It is best to shy away from toys containing plastic.*

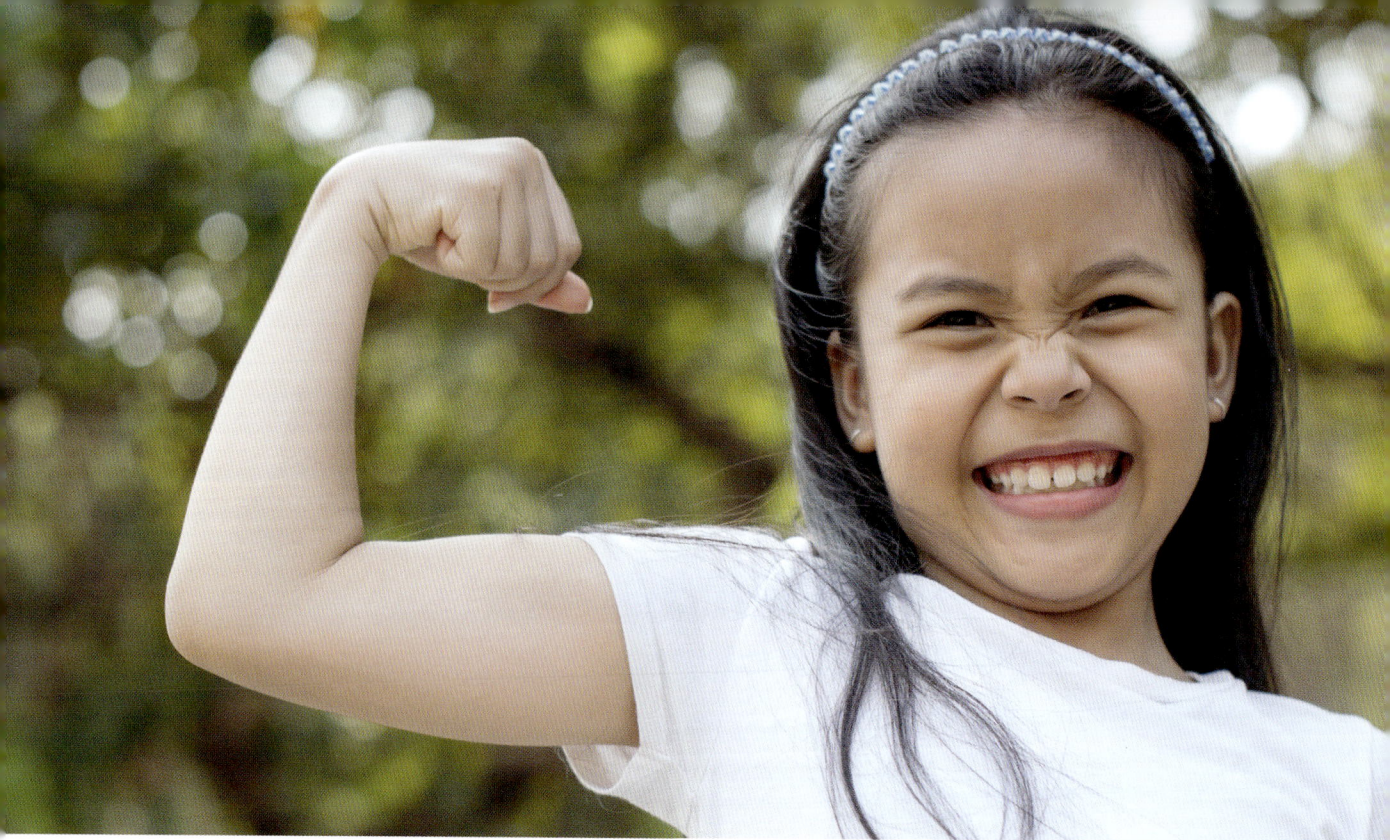

Chapter Ten: Safety Tips

"When to step in and when to step out is a fundamental parenting question.... At the same time that we want children to build skills and confidence, we also want to ensure that they are safe." — **Judy Frizlen**[386]

For new parents, few things seem more important than safety. Most parents are endowed with an intuitive sense of what is best for their little ones. In addition, there are some common precautions that can be useful in keeping children safe.

In this chapter, we will:

- Describe steps parents can take to babyproof their home
- Note considerations regarding car seats and strollers
- Review choking and chemical hazards

Babyproofing the Home

Admittedly, a newborn will not be crawling around the house on day one. Nevertheless, it is prudent to prepare early on for the day when a baby becomes mobile and begins exploring their environment. A few simple steps can go a long way toward making the home a safer place for children as they begin to crawl and eventually to walk. Taking these steps early on will provide peace of

> *It is prudent to prepare early on for the day when a baby...begins exploring their environment.*

mind that a child will be as safe as possible in the home as they develop.

Covering electrical outlets is an inexpensive and effective intervention to prevent electric shocks. Outlet covers are readily available at stores and online. They should cover any outlet that is at floor level or may be accessible to a young child.

Another precaution is to identify furniture with sharp corners and either remove the item or place padded covers over the corners. All children will fall and get bumps and bruises as they begin to stand up and learn to walk, but parents can minimize serious injuries by covering particularly hazardous edges.

At some point in toddlerhood, a child will begin to climb, turning the living room or other rooms in the house into a jungle gym. Securing furniture such as bookcases or dressers to the wall can prevent them from falling over and crushing a child.

Parents will additionally want to be cognizant of suffocation risks (for example, from plastic bags) or items that may pose a risk of strangulation, such as cords for blinds or any materials that a child could potentially wrap around their neck. Parents can minimize risks by placing these items out of reach or removing them from areas where a child may be able to access them.

Last, gates or barriers that obstruct access to stairs, pools, and water are safety features that can prevent falls or drowning.

> *Outlet covers are readily available at stores and online.*

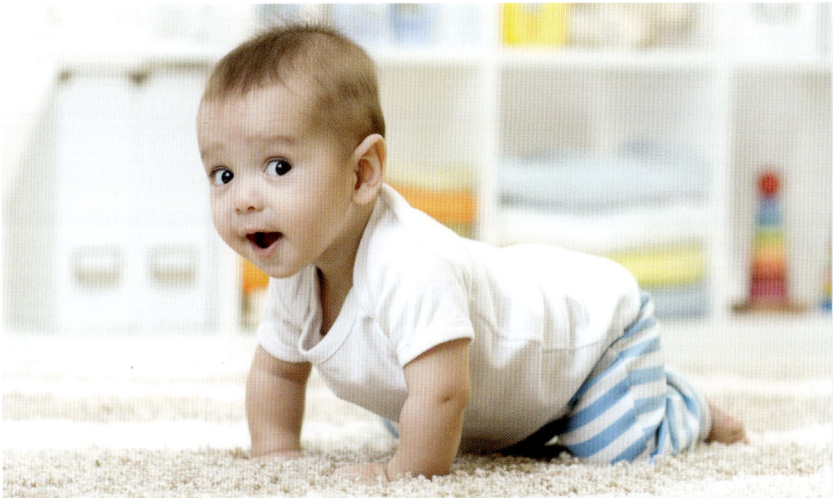

© Oksana Kuzmina/Adobe Stock

Car Seats and Strollers

Before the birth of a child, it is important to select a safe car seat for the drive home from the hospital or trips around town. Given the wide variety of car seats available, it can be difficult to decide which is best. Considerations may include selecting a car seat that is nontoxic and ensuring that the seat is designed for infants. Some car seats are infant-only, while convertible or adjustable car seats are designed to accommodate children as they grow.

It is important that infant car seats be rear-facing and installed in the back seat. Follow the manufacturer's weight recommendations to maximize safety benefits. Local fire departments often provide car seat installation for parents who want to ensure that they have installed a seat properly. The National Highway Traffic Safety Administration offers more information about car seats at its website.[387] Newer cars include tethers and latches that make increased safety easier.

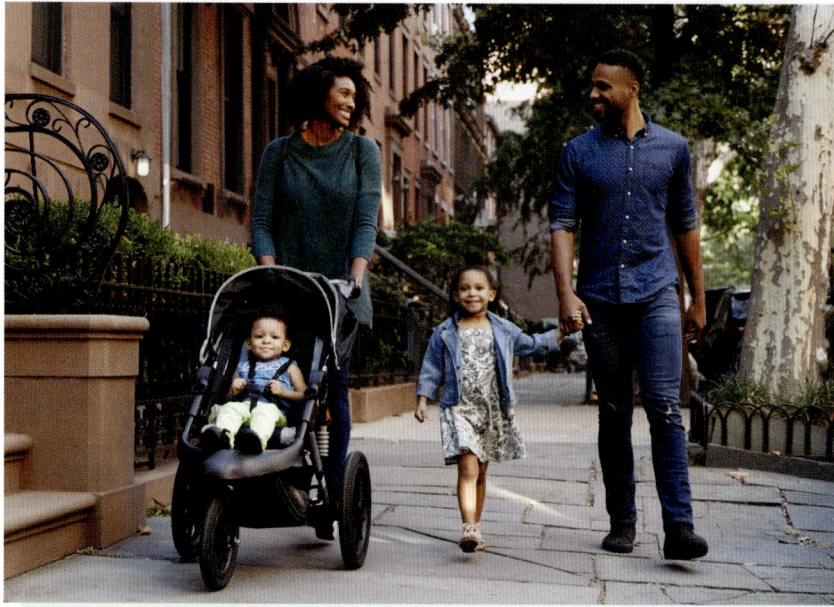

© Monkey Business/Adobe Stock

Many parents purchase strollers so they can get out and about with their newborn. When shopping for a stroller, parents need to make sure it is appropriate for infants and fits the family's lifestyle. In the first two to four months, infants do not have the ability to hold their heads up, so a stroller should be able to recline enough that the baby's head can rest back comfortably. Additional stroller safety features include the brake placement and wheel width. Parents should be able to apply the brakes with ease, and the stroller should be stable on uneven surfaces.

> *It is important that infant car seats be rear-facing and installed in the back seat.*

Choking and Accidental Ingestion

Few things are more terrifying than a young child choking.[388] Choking occurs when food or a foreign object obstructs the airway and causes suffocation. When children begin exploring by putting objects in their mouths and start eating solid foods, choking can become more of a concern.

The main thing parents can do to prevent choking is to keep small objects out of a little one's reach. Additionally, parents can keep their child's mouth occupied by providing toys designed to be chewed on that do not pose a choking hazard.

When a child transitions to solid foods, parents should make sure to cut pieces of food to a size that the child can easily swallow if they forget to chew. Always monitor children during mealtimes to ensure safety and be there to assist if needed. If choking does occur, parents should know the Heimlich maneuver, which can help remove the obstruction. To learn the proper technique, check for local infant first-aid courses or review online resources.

If a child swallows a foreign object such as a coin or small toy, contact a health care provider immediately for guidance. The Mayo Clinic offers more information on choking at its website.[389]

Other Potential Child Hazards

Another potential child hazard are dangerous cleaning agents, medications, cosmetics, and other chemical-containing products. The first line of defense for preventing this danger is to store these products in an area inaccessible to the child.

If a child does come into contact with a dangerous substance, the first thing to do is call Poison Control (reachable 24 hours a day at 800-222-1222) or emergency services for guidance. It used to be common practice to induce vomiting, but we now know that some products can cause additional harm while being evacuated. By quickly contacting a poison control expert, parents will learn what steps to take to keep their child safe and healthy.

> *The main thing parents can do to prevent choking is to keep small objects out of a little one's reach.*

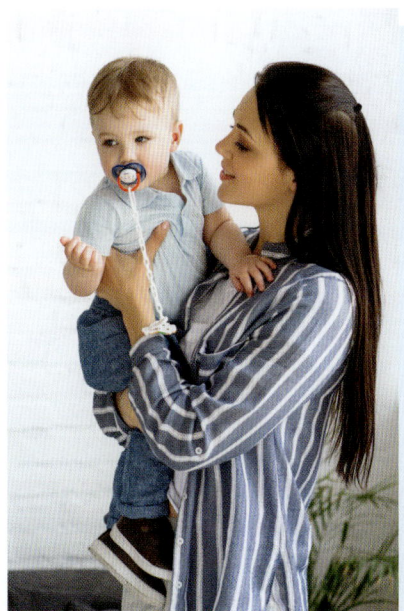

© LIGHTFIELD STUDIOS/Adobe Stock

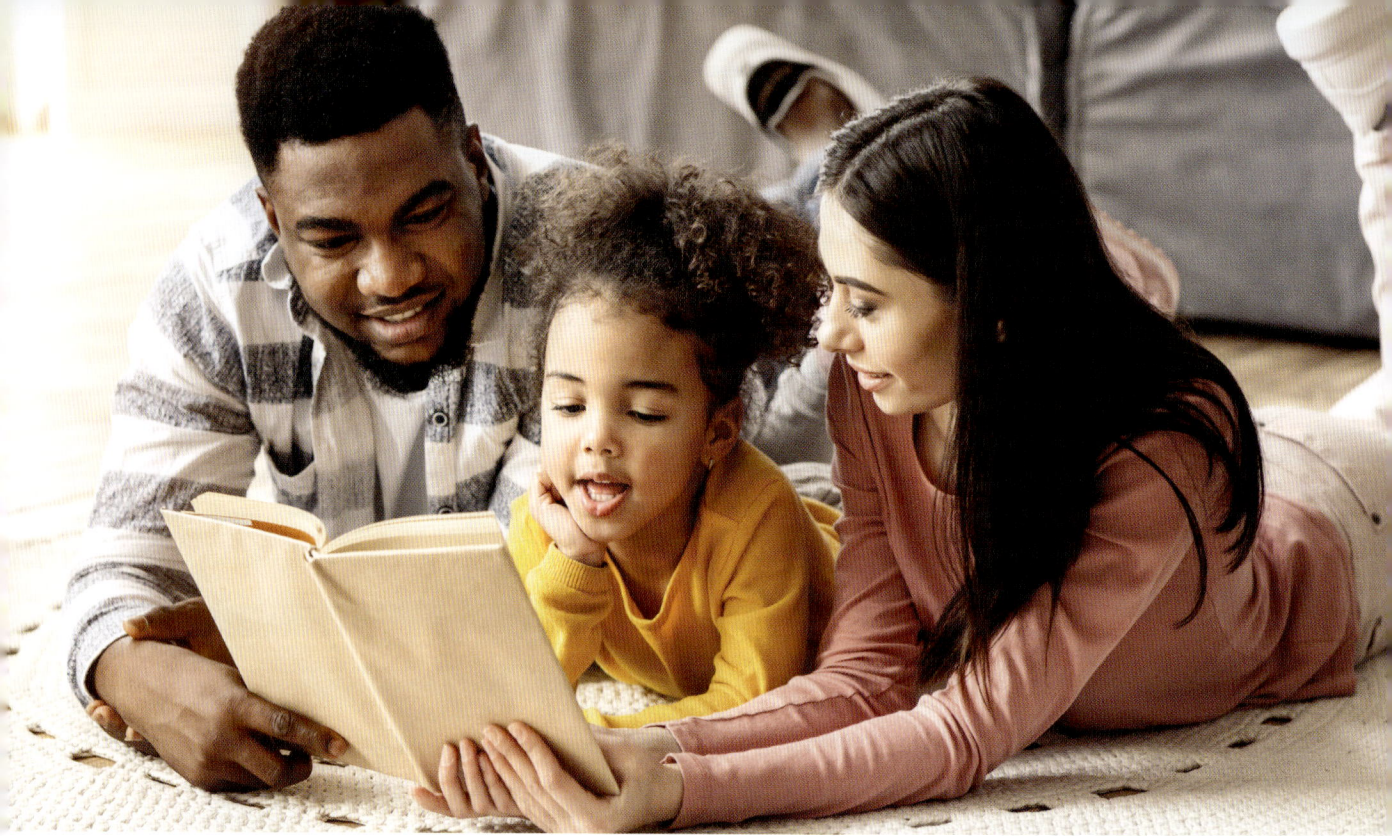

Chapter Eleven: The Parenting Journey

"Parenting is too important not to enjoy it." — **Simplicity Parenting website**[390]

Becoming a parent is a time of great change—it's joyous and exciting, but it can also be disruptive and stressful. From experiencing lack of sleep to balancing relationships, employment, child care, and leisure activities, many transitions take place when a new child arrives. Although each person's experience will be different, it is prudent to anticipate the challenges that may arise with caring for a newborn and have strategies in place to optimize health and well-being.

Wellness, according to one definition, is a holistic, all-encompassing concept with eight separate dimensions—physical, social, emotional, spiritual, intellectual, vocational, financial, and environmental.[391] Depending on parents' circumstances, having a new child won't necessarily affect all of these areas. At the same time, however, these dimensions often overlap and may influence each other, as when something affects a person not only physically but also emotionally (and vice versa).

> *It is prudent to anticipate the challenges that may arise with caring for a newborn.*

In this chapter, we will:

- Touch on a few of the most salient disruptions which may occur in the early stages of parenthood
- Suggest coping strategies to help during the first few months of a child's life

Sleep

Adequate sleep is vital for good health.[392] Sleep deprivation can have a detrimental effect on the immune system, mood, and cognitive function. Newborns typically wake every two to three hours for feedings, which means the mothers or parents are usually up every two to three hours as well, particularly if the baby is breastfeeding. Mothers of newborns will likely not be sleeping through the night.

Although nothing can be done about this unfortunate aspect of caring for a newborn, there are a few things that can help mothers get through this phase. Per one researcher, newborns sleep approximately 14 to 20 hours a day.[393] To the extent that other responsibilities allow, mothers can nap while their baby sleeps, allowing them to catch up on sleep and avoid some of the pitfalls of sleep deprivation.

Mothers also can lean on their spouse/partner or other support persons in the home, if available, to help with night-time diaper changes or, if the child is bottle-feeding, with feedings. Ultimately, a mother's best friend is time—as children develop, they will sleep for longer intervals. Many children sleep through the night by six months of age. Until then, families will need to experiment to figure out the strategies that work best for them.

> **Many children sleep through the night by six months of age.**

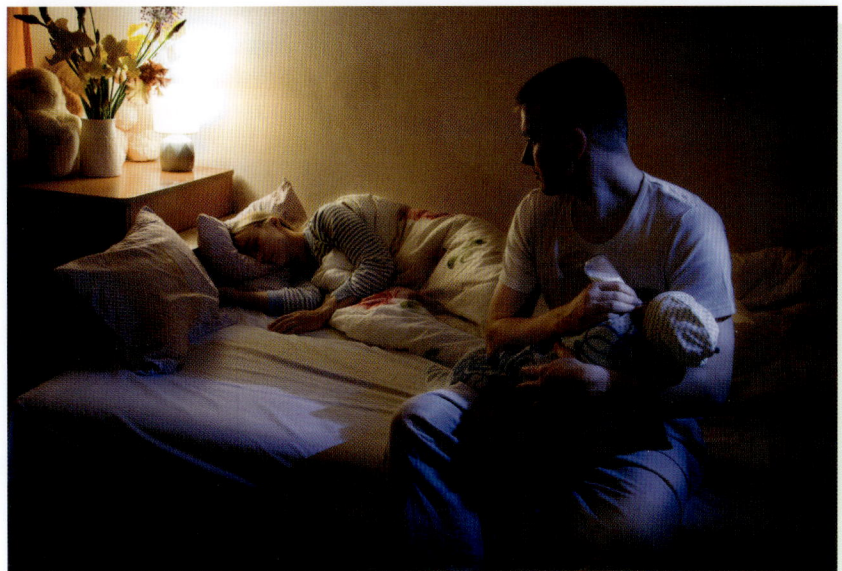

© Marina/Adobe Stock

Exercise

It's no secret that exercise is integral to physical and mental health. Though most new mothers will not be ready to run a marathon after giving birth, incorporating light exercise into their daily routine can help them stay healthy and grounded. On the other hand, increased postpartum bleeding can be a sign of too much physical activity. Mothers should consult with a health care provider before beginning any new exercise regime.

Walking and stretching are great ways to stay active and ease back into other forms of physical activity without risk of over-exertion. Research also indicates that postpartum physical activities like walking and stretching promote cardiovascular health and weight loss, and reduce the incidence of depression and anxiety.[394]

Many areas offer exercise classes designed for new mothers and their babies. These group classes may be a good option for those who enjoy a motivational and social atmosphere.

Postpartum Nutrition

In addition to exercise, consuming nutritious food is a great way for a mother to maintain her health during the postpartum period. Whole, unprocessed foods contain the most nutrients. Conversely, processed foods, including fast food and frozen meals, lack nutrients and contain high levels of unhealthy vegetable oils, refined sugars, and chemical additives. The Weston A. Price Foundation's article titled "Nourishing the New Mother: The Lost Art of Postpartum Care" offers an extensive discussion of the importance of "deep nutrition" during the postpartum period.[395]

Planning and preparing meals before delivery can help ensure parents will have healthy, nutritious meals on hand. Cooking and freezing meals in advance or receiving meals from a support network are strategies a new mother can use to reduce her burden after birth, helping her to maintain adequate nutrition while she establishes new routines.

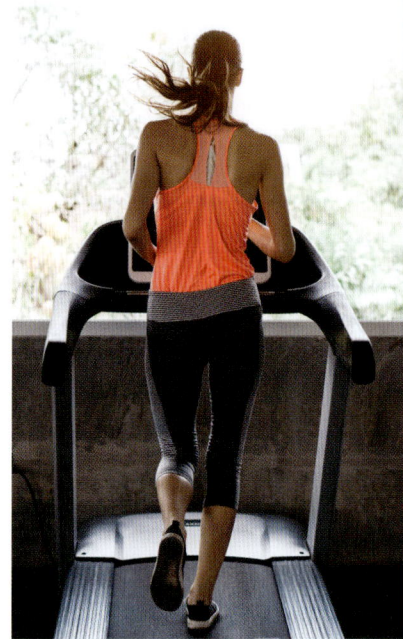

© WS Films/Adobe Stock

Mothers should consult with a health care provider before beginning any new exercise regime.

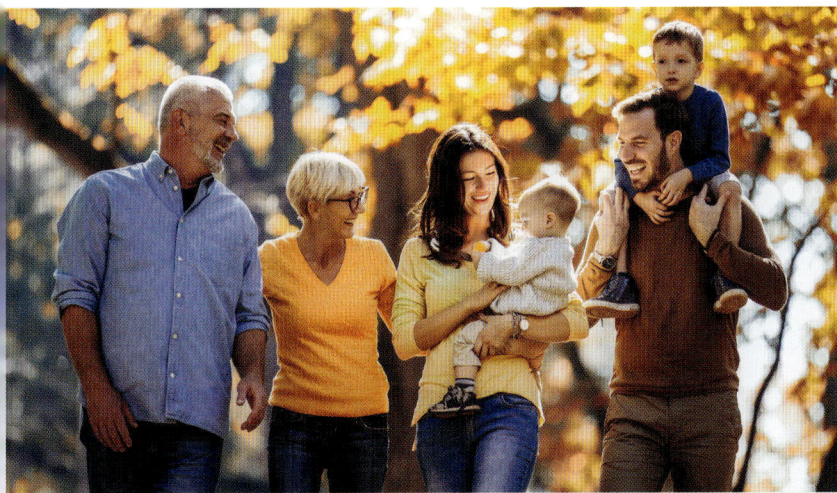

© Mediteraneo/Adobe Stock

Everyone will feel differently and find their own ways of navigating the first months of parenthood.

Social Support

Strong social support is another important element of maintaining overall wellness during the postpartum period. Having a network of family and friends to lean on can help with all aspects of the newborn period. From helping with shopping, meals, and cleaning to caring for other children, social support is indispensable.

The aforementioned suggestions regarding exercise and nutrition will be easier to implement when others are there for support. That said, not everyone is in a situation where family or close friends are nearby. If this is the case, communicating with loved ones remotely may provide moral support and give mothers and fathers a sounding board when they are feeling stressed or tired.

A Journey

Everyone will feel differently and find their own ways of navigating the first months of parenthood. It can be helpful for parents to reflect on what they value most—ranging from relationships to leisure activities—and brainstorm strategies for maintaining some of these priorities. Considering what is realistic and planning early on can aid parents in achieving optimum wellness during this life transition and help set them on a strong footing for their journey into parenthood.

Appendix: Typical Developmental Milestones, 2 Months Through 4 Years of Age

TYPE OF MILESTONE	2 MONTHS OF AGE
Social/Emotional	• Develops ability to briefly self-calm by bringing hands to mouth and sucking on hands • May begin to smile at people • Begins to look at parents' faces
Language/ Communication	• Develops ability to coo • May make gurgling sounds • Starts to turn head toward sounds
Cognitive (Learning, Thinking, Problem-Solving)	• May learn to pay attention to faces • May begin to follow things with eyes • May recognize people at a distance • Begins to act bored and cry or fuss if an activity does not change quickly enough
Movement/Physical Development	• May be able to hold head up • May begin to push up when lying on tummy • Leg and arm movements may become smoother

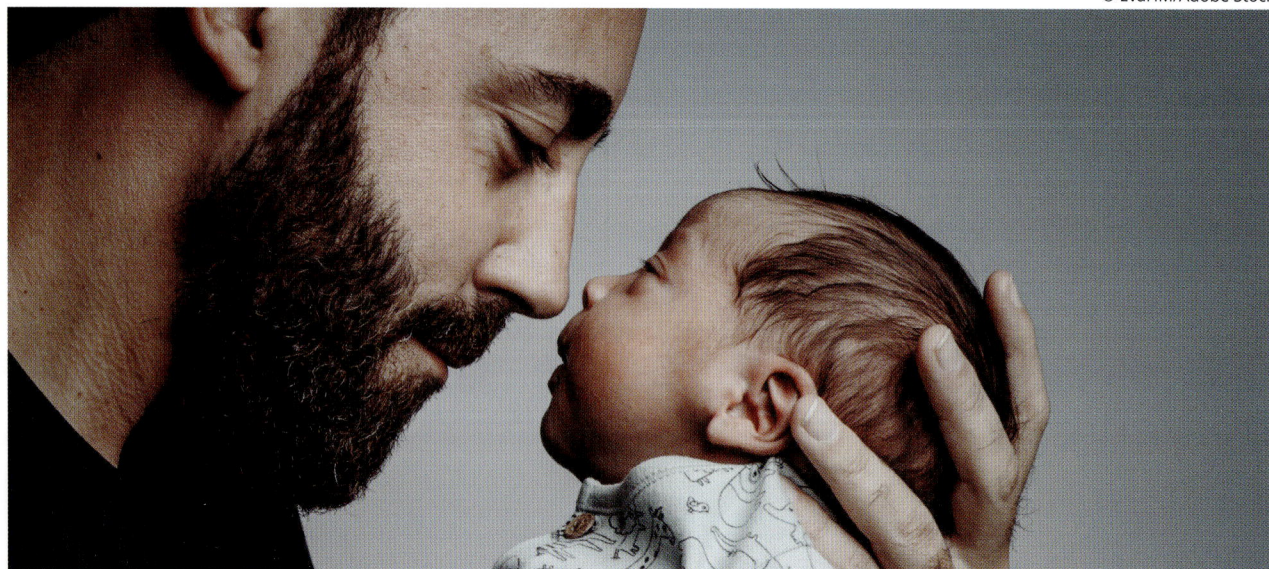

TYPE OF MILESTONE	4 MONTHS OF AGE
Social/Emotional	• May smile spontaneously—especially at people • May be able to copy some movements and facial expressions such as smiling and frowning • Enjoys playing with people (and may cry when the playing ends)
Language/ Communication	• Able to babble with expression • Able to copy sounds they hear • Learns to cry in different ways to convey hunger, pain, or fatigue
Cognitive (Learning, Thinking, Problem-Solving)	• Able to indicate happiness or sadness • Able to respond to affection • May reach for a toy with one hand • Uses hands and eyes together in coordination—such as seeing a toy and reaching for it • Can follow moving things with their eyes from side to side • Can watch faces closely • Recognizes familiar people and things at a distance
Movement/Physical Development	• Able to hold head steady with no support • May push down on legs when feet are on a hard surface • May be able to roll over from tummy to back • Can hold a toy and shake it • Can swing at dangling toys • Brings hands to mouth • Can push up on elbows when lying on stomach

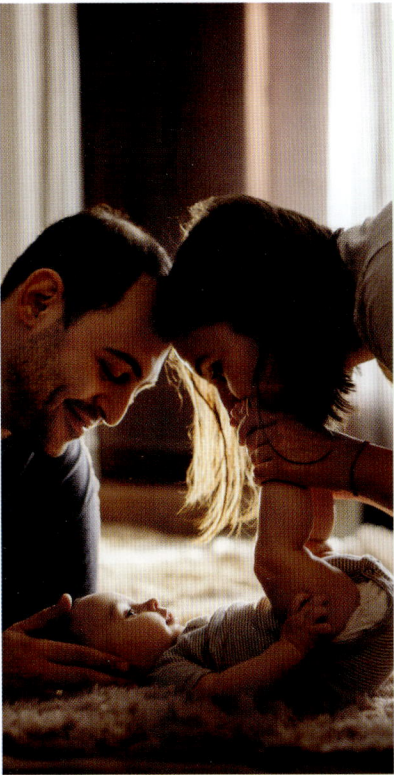

© Olga Ternavskaya/Adobe Stock

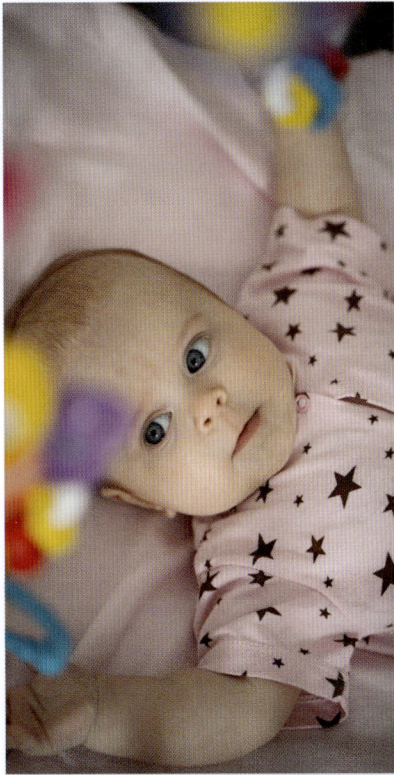

© Evgenia Tiplyashina/Adobe Stock

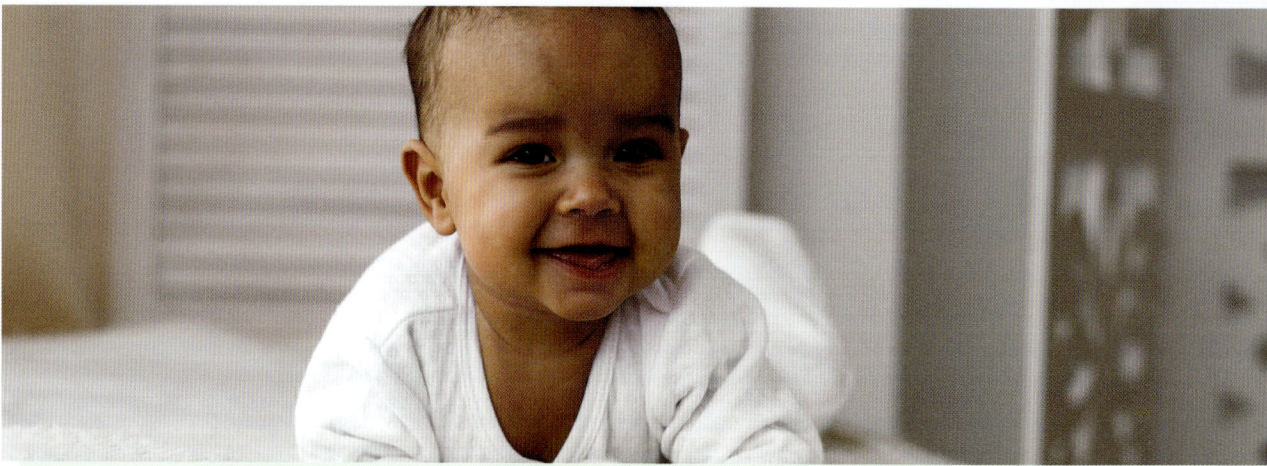

TYPE OF MILESTONE	6 MONTHS OF AGE
Social/Emotional	• May learn to recognize familiar faces and know if someone is a stranger • Likes to play with others—especially their parents • Responds to other people's emotions • Often seems happy • Develops a desire to look at self in a mirror
Language/ Communication	• Responds to sounds by making sounds • Can string vowels together when babbling ("ah," "eh," "oh") • Likes taking turns with parents while making sounds • Begins to respond to own name • Makes sounds to show joy and displeasure • Begins to say consonant sounds (jabbering with "m," "b")
Cognitive (Learning, Thinking, Problem-Solving)	• May look around at things nearby • May show curiosity about things and try to get things that are out of reach • Brings things to mouth • Begins to pass things from one hand to the other
Movement/Physical Development	• May roll over in both directions (front to back and back to front) • When standing, legs can support weight • May be able to bounce • Begins to be able to sit without support • Can rock back and forth • Will sometimes crawl backwards before moving forward

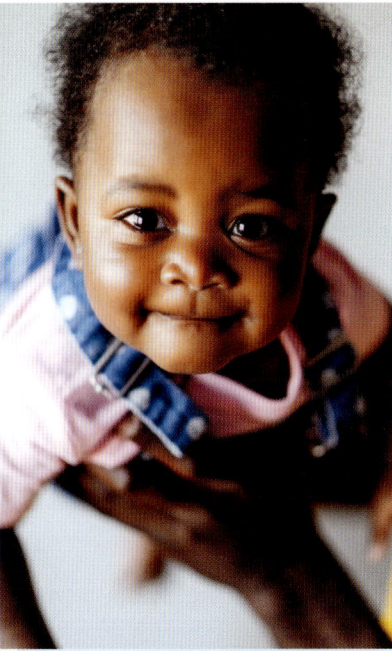
© Oscar Stock/Adobe Stock

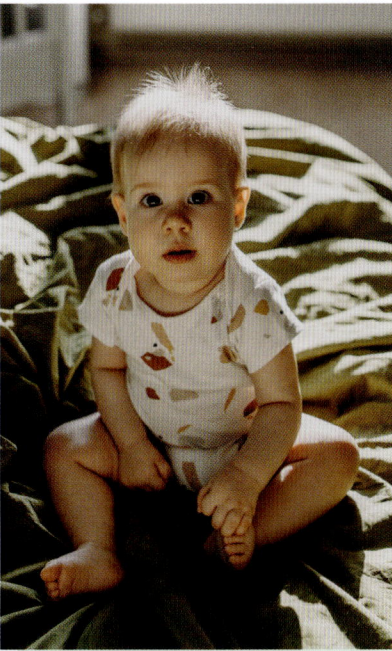
© Bostan Natalia/Adobe Stock

TYPE OF MILESTONE	9 MONTHS OF AGE
Social/Emotional	• Becomes afraid of strangers • May cling to familiar adults • Chooses favorite toys
Language/ Communication	• Can understand the meaning of "No" • Can make a variety of different sounds (e.g., "ma-ma-ma," "ba-ba-ba") • Can copy sounds and gestures of others • Uses fingers to point at things
Cognitive (Learning, Thinking, Problem-Solving)	• Will watch the path of something as it falls • Will look for things they see their parents hide • Can play peek-a-boo • Will put things in mouth
Movement/Physical Development	• May be able to stand while holding on to something or someone • Can pull up to a standing position • Can get into a sitting position • Can sit without support • Can crawl • Can move things smoothly from one hand to the other • Can pick up things like cereal O's between thumb and index finger

TYPE OF MILESTONE	1 YEAR OF AGE
Social/Emotional	• May be shy or nervous with strangers • May cry when parents leave • Chooses favorite things and people • May demonstrate fear in some situations • Will hand parents a book when wanting to hear a story • Will repeat sounds or actions to get attention • Will put out arms or legs to solicit help with getting dressed • May play games such as peek-a-boo or pat-a-cake
Language/ Communication	• Can respond to simple spoken requests • Can use simple gestures such as shaking head to mean "no" or waving to indicate "goodbye" • Can change verbal tone • Can say "mama" and "dada" and exclamations such as "uh-oh" • Will try to parrot words said by parents
Cognitive (Learning, Thinking, Problem-Solving)	• May learn to explore objects in different ways such as through shaking, banging, or throwing • May find hidden things more easily • May be able to choose the right picture or thing when it is named • May copy gestures • Will put things in and take things out of a container • Will start to use objects for their correct purpose, such as drinking out of a cup or brushing hair with a brush • May let things go without help • Can follow simple directions such as a request to pick up a toy
Movement/Physical Development	• May be able to pull up to stand • May be able to stand up alone • May be able to walk holding on to furniture • May be able to take a few steps without holding on to anything or anyone • May bang two things together • May poke people with index finger

TYPE OF MILESTONE	18 MONTHS OF AGE
Social/Emotional	• May like to hand things to others • May have temper tantrums • May be afraid of strangers • May show affection to familiar people • Likes to play simple pretend games such as feeding a doll • May cling to a caregiver in a new situation • May point to show others something of interest • May be willing to explore new spaces alone with parents close by
Language/ Communication	• May have the ability to say several single words • May shake head and say "no" • Will show someone something they want
Cognitive (Learning, Thinking, Problem-Solving)	• May be able to recognize what ordinary things are for (such as a phone, brush, or spoon) • May point to several body parts • May pretend to feed and care for a doll or a stuffed animal • May point to get the attention of others • May scribble on their own • Follows one-step verbal commands without any gestures
Movement/Physical Development	• May be able to walk alone • May walk up steps and run • Can pull toys while walking • Can help get undressed • Can drink from a cup • Can eat with a spoon

TYPE OF MILESTONE	2 YEARS OF AGE
Social/Emotional	• May copy others—especially adults and older children • May get excited when with other children • Will demonstrate more independence • May show defiant behavior and deliberately do things told not to do • Will play mainly beside other children (parallel playing), but may also begin to include other children in chase games
Language/ Communication	• May be able to point to things or pictures when named • May know the names of familiar people or body parts • Can say sentences with two to four words • Can follow simple instructions • Can repeat words overheard in conversation • Can point to things in a book
Cognitive (Learning, Thinking, Problem-Solving)	• May be able to find things when hidden, even under two or three covers • Can begin to sort shapes and colors • Can complete sentences and rhymes from familiar books • Can play simple make-believe games • Can build towers with four or more blocks • Can choose to use one hand more than the other • Can follow two-step instructions such as "pick up your shoes and put them in the closet" • Can name items in a picture book such as cat, bird, or dog
Movement/Physical Development	• May be able to stand on tiptoes • Can kick a ball • Can begin to run • Can walk up and down stairs holding on to something • Can climb onto and down from furniture without help • Can throw a ball overhead • Can make or copy straight lines and circles

TYPE OF MILESTONE	3 YEARS OF AGE
Social/Emotional	• May be able to copy adults and friends • May show affection for friends without prompting • May be willing to take turns in games • Will demonstrate empathy for a crying friend • Can get dressed and undressed • Understands the idea of "mine" and "his" or "hers" • Will reveal a wide range of emotions • Separation from parents becomes easier • May be upset by major changes in routine
Language/ Communication	• May be able to follow instructions with two or three steps • Can name most familiar things • May understand words such as "in," "on," and "under" • Can say first name, age, and sex • Can name a friend • Can talk well enough for strangers to understand most of the time • Can say words such as "I," "me," "we," "you," and some plurals • Can carry on a conversation using two to three sentences
Cognitive (Learning, Thinking, Problem-Solving)	• May be able to work toys with buttons, levers, and moving parts • Can play make-believe with dolls, animals, and people • Can work puzzles with three or four pieces • Can understand what "two" means • Can copy a circle with a pencil or crayon • Can turn book pages one at a time • Can build towers with more than six blocks • Can screw and unscrew jar lids and turn door handles
Movement/Physical Development	• May be able to climb well • Can run easily • Can pedal a tricycle • Can walk up and down stairs with one foot on each step

TYPE OF MILESTONE	4 YEARS OF AGE
Social/Emotional	• May enjoy doing new things • May become more creative in make-believe playing • Would rather play with other children than alone • Learns to cooperate with other children • Enjoys mimicking "Mommy" and "Daddy" • Often can't tell what is real and what is make-believe • Will talk about likes and interests
Language/ Communication	• Will enjoy telling stories • Can sing a song or recite a poem from memory, such as "Itsy Bitsy Spider" or "Wheels on the Bus" • Will understand some basic rules of grammar, such as correct use of "he" or "she" • Can say first and last name
Cognitive (Learning, Thinking, Problem-Solving)	• Can name some colors and numbers • Understands the idea of counting • Begins to understand the concept of time • Can remember the parts of a story • Understands the idea of "same" and "different" • Can draw a person with two to four body parts • Can use scissors • Can start to copy capital letters • Can play board and card games • Can predict what may happen next in a book
Movement/Physical Development	• Can hop and stand on one foot for up to two seconds at a time • Can pour, cut with supervision, and mash food • Can catch a bounced ball most of the time

Source: Dawn Lee Garzon et al., *Burns' Pediatric Primary Care*, 7th Edition, Elsevier, 2019.

Endnotes

1 Kathi J. Kemper, *The Holistic Pediatrician, Twentieth Anniversary Revised Edition: A Pediatrician's Comprehensive Guide to Safe and Effective Therapies for the 25 Most Common Ailments of Infants, Children, and Adolescents*, Harper Paperbacks, 2016.

2 John Thomson, Rahima Baldwin, Tim Kahn, Mildred Masheder, Lynne Oldfield, Dr. Michaela Glockler, and Roland Meighan, *Natural Childhood: The First Practical and Holistic Guide for Parents of the Developing Child*, Simon & Schuster, 1995.

3 Aviva Jill Romm. *Naturally Healthy Babies and Children: A Commonsense Guide to Herbal Remedies, Nutrition, and Health* (12th ed.), Celestial Arts, 2003.

4 "All About Birth & Primal Health," Birthing the Future, accessed Jan. 29, 2023, birthingthefuture.org/about-birthing.

5 "What Is Infertility?" Centers for Disease Control and Prevention, accessed Mar. 1, 2022, cdc.gov/reproductivehealth/features/what-is-infertility/index.html.

6 Veronica Tilden, "Restoring Male Fertility," Weston A. Price Foundation, Feb. 2, 2017, westonaprice.org/health-topics/mens-health/restoring-male-fertility/.

7 Randine Lewis, *The Infertility Cure: The Ancient Chinese Wellness Program for Getting Pregnant and Having Healthy Babies*, Little, Brown Spark, 2005.

8 Tilden, 2017.

9 "Find a Holistic Practitioner," Alternatives for Healing, accessed Dec. 28, 2022, alternativesforhealing.com/find-a-practitioner.

10 Resolve, The National Infertility Association, accessed Aug. 1, 2023, resolve.org.

11 Tilden, 2017.

12 Jorge E. Chavarro et al., "Dietary Fatty Acid Intakes and the Risk of Ovulatory Infertility," *The American Journal of Clinical Nutrition* 85, no. 1 (2007): 231–237, doi.org/10.1093/ajcn/85.1.231.

13 Kim Schuette, "Recovery from the Birth Control Pill & Other Hormonal Contraceptives," Weston A. Price Foundation, Aug. 15, 2016, westonaprice.org/health-topics/womens-health/recovery-birth-control-pill-hormonal-contraceptives.

14 Saba Shahin, Surya Pal Singh, and Chandra Mohini Chaturvedi, "Mobile Phone (1800MHz) Radiation Impairs Female Reproduction in Mice, *Mus musculus*, Through Stress Induced Inhibition of Ovarian and Uterine Activity," *Reproductive Toxicology* 73 (2017): 41–60, doi: 10.1016/j.reprotox.2017.08.001.

15 Lloyd Burrell, "Can Cell Phones Cause Female Infertility?", ElectricSense, Jan. 13, 2018, electricsense.com/cell-phones-female-infertility.

16 Tilden, 2017.

17 Aviva Romm, "Should You Detox Before Getting Pregnant?", Avivaromm.com, accessed Jan. 30, 2023, avivaromm.com/detox-before-getting-pregnant.

18 Tom P. Fleming et al., "Adaptive Responses of the Embryo to Maternal Diet and Consequences for Post-Implantation Development," *Reproduction, Fertility and Development* 24, no. 1 (2011): 35–44, doi.org/10.1071/RD11905.

19 Christopher Masterjohn, "Vitamins for Fetal Development: Conception to Birth," Weston A. Price Foundation, Jul. 23, 2013, westonaprice.org/health-topics/childrens-health/vitamins-for-fetal-development-conception-to-birth.

20 Sally Fallon Morell, "How to Have a Healthy Pregnancy," Wise Traditions Podcast Episode 284, Dec. 7, 2020, westonaprice.org/podcast/how-to-have-a-healthy-pregnancy.

21 Mark McAfee, "Is Raw Milk Safe," Wise Traditions Podcast Episode 151, Sep. 10, 2018, westonaprice.org/podcast/151-is-raw-milk-safe.

22 Sally Fallon and Mary G. Enig, "Be Kind to Your Grains ... and Your Grains Will Be Kind to You," Weston A. Price Foundation, Jan. 1, 2000, westonaprice.org/health-topics/food-features/be-kind-to-your-grains-and-your-grains-will-be-kind-to-you.

23 Morell, "How to Have a Healthy Pregnancy," 2020.

24 Sabina Bastos Maia et al., "Vitamin A and Pregnancy: A Narrative Review," *Nutrients* 11, no. 3 (2019): 681, doi: 10.3390/nu11030681.

25 N.E. Buss et al., "The Teratogenic Metabolites of Vitamin A in Women Following Supplements and Liver," *Human & Experimental Toxicology* 13, no. 1 (1994): 33–43, doi: 10.1177/096032719401300106.

26 "Vitamin A Palmitate: Avoid Synthetic Isolates Whenever Possible!", The Health Coach, 2012, thehealthcoach1.com/?p=1640.

27 Masterjohn, 2013.

28 Sandrine Perez, "What About Prenatal Vitamins?", *Nourishing Our Children*, accessed Jan. 30, 2023, nourishingourchildren.org/2014/07/06/what-about-prenatal-vitamins.

29 Sally Fallon Morell, "Diet for Pregnant and Nursing Mothers," Weston A. Price Foundation, Jan. 10, 2004, westonaprice.org/health-topics/diet-for-pregnant-and-nursing-mothers.

30 Masterjohn, 2013.

31 "10 Thousand Chemicals in Food and Food Packaging: What Are These Substances Doing to Our Children," Children's Health Defense, Aug. 23, 2018, childrenshealthdefense.org/news/10-thousand-chemicals-in-food-and-food-packaging-what-are-these-substances-doing-to-our-children.

32 Jessica A. Grieger et al., "Pre-pregnancy Fast Food and Fruit Intake Is Associated with Time to Pregnancy," *Human Reproduction* 33, no. 6 (2018): 1063–1070, doi.org/10.1093/humrep/dey079.

33 Chavarro et al., 2007.

34 Razieh Farzad and Jeanette Andrade, "Selenium and Mercury Toxicity: the Tale of Fish," University of Florida/IFAS Extension, publication #FSHN22-4, Feb. 21, 2022, edis.ifas.ufl.edu/publication/FS437.

35 Jessica A. Grieger, "Preconception Diet, Fertility, and Later Health in Pregnancy," *Current Opinion in Obstetrics and Gynecology* 32, no. 3 (2020): 227–232, doi: 10.1097/GCO.0000000000000629.

36 Jim Earles, "Sugar-Free Blues: Everything You Wanted to Know About Artificial Sweeteners," Weston A. Price Foundation, Feb. 19, 2004, westonaprice.org/health-topics/modern-foods/sugar-free-blues-everything-you-wanted-to-know-about-artificial-sweeteners.

37 Gail Elbek, "Why Babies Should Not Be Fed Soy: Testimony to the CERHR Soy Infant Formula Panel," Weston A. Price Foundation, Feb. 10, 2010, westonaprice.org/health-topics/soy-alert/why-babies-should-not-be-fed-soy.

38 Jan Gill, "The Effects of Moderate Alcohol Consumption on Female Hormone Levels and Reproductive Function," *Alcohol and Alcoholism* 35, no. 5 (2000): 417–423, doi.org/10 .1093/alcalc/35.5.417.

39 Jan Eggert, Holger Theobald, and Peter Engfeldt, "Effects of Alcohol Consumption on Female Fertility During an 18-Year Period," *Fertility and Sterility* 81, no. 2 (2004): 379–383, doi.org/10.1016/j.fertnstert.2003.06 .018.

40 Andrea Sansone et al., "Smoke, Alcohol and Drug Addiction and Male Fertility," *Reproductive Biology and Endocrinology* 16, no. 1 (2018):3, doi: 10.1186/s12958-018-0320-7.

41 Josie M.L. McConnell and Linda Petrie, "Mitochondrial DNA Turnover Occurs During Preimplantation Development and Can Be Modulated by Environmental Factors," *Reproductive Biomedicine Online* 9, no. 4 (2004): 418–424, doi: 10.1016 /s1472-6483(10)61277-1.

42 Joseph Pizzorno. "Environmental Toxins and Infertility," *Integrative Medicine (Encinitas)* 17, no. 2 (2018): 8–11, pubmed.ncbi.nlm.nih.gov /30962779.

43 Katherine Gillespie, "The 10 Best Natural Cleaning Products," *The Strategist*, updated Aug. 10, 2022, nymag.com/strategist/article/best -natural-organic-cleaning-products .html.

44 Konstantinos Douros et al., "Prenatal Maternal Stress and the Risk of Asthma in Children," *Frontiers in Pediatrics* 5 (2017): 202, doi.org/10 .3389/fped.2017.00202.

45 "How Stress During Pregnancy Affects Your Baby," *Exploring your mind*, updated Feb. 10, 2019, exploringyourmind.com/stress -during-pregnancy-affects-baby.

46 Abbey Kruper et al., "How to Manage Stress Naturally During Pregnancy," *Society of Behavioral Medicine*, accessed Dec. 30, 2022, sbm.org/healthy-living /how-to-manage-stress-naturally -during-pregnancy.

47 Alice D. Domar and Sheila Curry Oakes, *Finding Calm for the Expectant Mom: Tools for Reducing Stress, Anxiety, and Mood Swings During Your Pregnancy*, TarcherPerigee, 2016.

48 Lynn Clark Callister and Inaam Khalaf, "Spirituality in Childbearing Women," *Journal of Perinatal Education* 19, no. 2 (2010): 16–24, doi.org/10 .1624/105812410x495514.

49 Jill C. Nienhiser, "Find Nutrient-Dense Foods," Weston A. Price Foundation, Jan. 26, 2012, westonaprice.org/find-nutrient-dense -foods.

50 Elizabeth Plourde, "Sunscreens: The Dark Side of Avoiding the Sun," Weston A. Price Foundation, Jan. 22, 2019, westonaprice.org/health-topics /environmental-toxins/sunscreens -the-dark-side-of-avoiding-the-sun.

51 Elizabeth Plourde, "Is the Sun to Blame? Or Is it the Sunscreen?", Wise Traditions Podcast Episode 374, Jul. 4, 2022, westonaprice.org/podcast/is -the-sun-to-blame-or-is-it-the -sunscreen.

52 James Lyons-Weiler, "Moms Were Right: Acetaminophen During Pregnancy Can Cause ADHD, Autism," *The Defender*, Nov. 15, 2022, childrenshealthdefense.org/defender /acetaminophen-pregnancy-adhd -autism-jlw.

53 Molly M. Lynch et al., "Making Decisions About Medication Use During Pregnancy: Implications for Communication Strategies," *Maternal and Child Health Journal* 22, no. 1 (2018): 92–100, doi: 10.1007/s10995 -017-2358-0.

54 Children's Health Defense Team, "Think the FDA Is Looking Out for Your Health? History Tells a Different Story," *The Defender*, Oct. 6, 2021, childrenshealthdefense.org/defender /fda-regulatory-capture-revolving -door-jobs.

55 Children's Health Defense Team, "Think the FDA Is Looking Out for Your Health?" 2021, childrenshealthdefense.org/defender /fda-regulatory-capture-revolving -door-jobs.

56 Leanna Skarnulis, "Toxins and Pregnancy," *WebMD*, Oct. 1, 2008, webmd.com/baby/features/pregnancy -and-toxins.

57 Julia Pletz, Francisco Sanchez-Bayo, and Henk A. 1onekes, "Dose-Response Analysis Indicating Time-Dependent Neurotoxicity Caused by Organic and Inorganic Mercury—Implications for Toxic Effects in the Developing Brain," *Toxicology* 347–349 (2016): 1–5, doi: 10.1016/j.tox .2016.02.006.

58 Centers for Disease Control and Prevention, "Updated Recommendations for Use of Tetanus Toxoid, Reduced Diphtheria Toxoid and Acellular Pertussis Vaccine (Tdap) in Pregnancy Women and Persons Who Have or Anticipate Having Close Contact with an Infant Aged <12 Months—Advisory Committee on Immunization Practices (ACIP), 2011," *Morbidity and Mortality Weekly Report* 60, no. 41 (2011): 1424–1426, PMID: 22012116, bit.ly/3rRBckt.

59 "Appendix B: Vaccines," Vaccine Excipient Table, Centers for Disease Control and Prevention, November 2021, cdc.gov/vaccines/pubs/pinkbook /downloads/appendices/appdx-full-b .pdf.

60 Elyse O. Kharbanda et al., "Receipt of Pertussis Vaccine During Pregnancy Across 7 Vaccine Safety Datalink Sites," *Preventive Medicine* 67 (2014): 316–319, doi: 10.1016/j .ypmed.2014.05.025.

61 Hilda Razzaghi et al., "Influenza and Tdap Vaccination Coverage Among Pregnant Women—United States, April 2020," *Morbidity and Mortality Weekly Report* 69, no. 39 (2020): 1391–1397, doi: 10.15585/mmwr.mm 6939a2.

62 Alisa Kachikis, Linda O. Eckert, and Janet Englund, "Who's the Target: Mother or Baby?", *Viral Immunology* 31, no. 2 (2018): 184–194, doi: 10 .1089/vim.2017.0135.

63 Nicole M. Smith et al., "Prevention and Control of Influenza," *Morbidity and Mortality Weekly Report* 55, no. RR-10 (2006): 1–42, PMID: 16874296, bit.ly/3DCJNdn.

64 Adacel, accessed Feb. 10, 2023, wayback.archive-it.org/7993 /20170723151948/www.fda.gov /downloads/BiologicsBloodVaccines /Vaccines/ApprovedProducts/UCM14 2764.pdf.

65 Adacel, accessed Feb. 10, 2023, fda .gov/media/119862/download.

66 World Health Organization, "Harmonized Approaches for the Vigilance of Interventions During Pregnancy," *Weekly Epidemiological Record* 93, no. 3 (2018): 28–30, apps .who.int/iris/bitstream/handle /10665/259874/WER9303.pdf;jsession id=95B5DC87BDDD921E4796E1ED6101 82C1?sequence=1.

67 "How to Implement Influenza Vaccination of Pregnant Women," World Health Organization, Jan. 1, 2016, who.int/publications/i/item /WHO-IVB-16.06.

68 "Reproductive Toxicity and Vaccines," *Children's Health Defense*, Apr. 20, 2018, childrenshealthdefense.org /government/fda/reproductive -toxicity-and-vaccines.

69 Center for Biologics Evaluation and Research, "Guidance for Industry: Considerations for Developmental Toxicity Studies for Preventive and Therapeutic Vaccines for Infectious Disease Indications," U.S. Department of Health and Human Services, Food and Drug Administration, February 2006, fda.gov/media/73986/download.

70 Paul Barrow, "Developmental and Reproductive Toxicity Testing of Vaccines," *Journal of Pharmacological and Toxicological Methods* 65, no. 2 (2012): 58–63, doi: 10.1016/j.vascn.2011.12.001.

71 Robert F. Kennedy, Jr., "CDC Study Shows Up to 7.7-fold Greater Odds of Miscarriage After Influenza Vaccine," Children's Health Defense, Sep. 19, 2017, childrenshealthdefense.org/news/cdc-study-shows-7-7-fold-greater-odds-miscarriage-influenza-vaccine.

72 Robert F. Kennedy, Jr. and Lyn Redwood, "Flu Shots During Pregnancy & Autism: Cause for Concern," Children's Health Defense, Dec. 23, 2016, childrenshealthdefense.org/news/flu-shots-pregnancy-autism-cause-concern.

73 "Flu Vaccine Facts: What You Need to Know for 2018-19," Children's Health Defense, Jan. 1, 2018, childrenshealthdefense.org/news/flu-vaccine-facts.

74 "About VigiBase," Uppsala Monitoring Centre, accessed Feb. 8, 2023, who-umc.org/vigibase.

75 Pathiyil Ravi Shankar, "VigiAccess: Promoting Public Access to VigiBase," *Indian Journal of Pharmacology* 48, no. 5 (2016): 606–607, doi: 10.4103/0253-7613.190766.

76 Children's Health Defense Team, "Flu Shots During Pregnancy Failed to Lower the Risk of Fetal Death, Preterm Birth and Low Birth Weight," Children's Health Defense, Aug. 6, 2019, childrenshealthdefense.org/news/flu-shots-during-pregnancy-failed-to-lower-the-risk-of-fetal-death-preterm-birth-and-low-birth-weight.

77 Buzz Hollander, "Pfizer's RSV Vaccine for Pregnant Women Is Heading for Approval," Buzz About Medicine, Substack, Nov. 4, 2022, doctorbuzz.substack.com/p/pfizers-rsv-vaccine-for-pregnant.

78 "COVID-19 Vaccines While Pregnant or Breastfeeding," Centers for Disease Control and Prevention, updated Oct. 20, 2022, cdc.gov/coronavirus/2019-ncov/vaccines/recommendations/pregnancy.html.

79 Children's Health Defense Team, "CDC Report Blames Pregnancy-Related Deaths on Heart, Mental Health Issues, But No Mention of Vaccines as Possible Risk Factor," *The Defender*, Sep. 23, 2022, childrenshealthdefense.org/defender/cdc-maternal-death-rate-heart-mental-health-vaccination-pregnancy.

80 "Guidelines for Vaccinating Pregnant Women," Centers for Disease Control and Prevention, accessed Feb. 8, 2023, cdc.gov/vaccines/pregnancy/hcp-toolkit/guidelines.html.

81 Children's Health Defense Team, "Who Benefits When Pharma-Funded FDA Fast-Tracks Drugs and Vaccines? Not Consumers, Critics Warn," *The Defender*, Oct. 13, 2022, childrenshealthdefense.org/defender/fda-big-pharma-drugs-vaccines-consumers/.

82 Alireza Ebrahimzadeh Bideskan et al., "Maternal Exposure to Titanium Dioxide Nanoparticles During Pregnancy and Lactation Alters Offspring Hippocampal mRNA BAX and Bcl-2 Levels, Induces Apoptosis and Decreases Neurogenesis," *Experimental and Toxicologic Pathology* 69, no. 6 (2017): 329–337, doi: 10.1016/j.etp.2017.02.006.

83 Sonia Ndeupen et al., "The mRNA-LNP Platform's Lipid Nanoparticle Component Used in Preclinical Vaccine Studies Is Highly Inflammatory," *iScience* 24, no. 12 (2021): 103479, doi: 10.1016/j.isci.2021.103479.

84 Sucharit Bhakdi, "Vaccine Ingredient Problems You Never Heard About" (Panel Discussion), in "Symposium 5, Session 1: The Fundamental Flaws of mRNA Vaccine Technology," Doctors for COVID Ethics, Jan. 20, 2023, doctors4covidethics.org/session-i-the-fundamental-flaws-of-mrna-vaccine-technology-2.

85 Xinran Li, Abdulaziz M. Aldayel, and Zhengrong Cui, "Aluminum Hydroxide Nanoparticles Show a Stronger Vaccine Adjuvant Activity than Traditional Aluminum Hydroxide Microparticles," *Journal of Controlled Release* 173 (2014): 148–157, doi: 10.1016/j.jconrel.2013.10.032.

86 Antonietta M. Gatti and Stefano Montanari, "New Quality-Control Investigations on Vaccines: Micro- and Nanocontamination," *International Journal of Vaccines & Vaccination* 4, no. 1 (2017), medcraveonline.com/IJVV/IJVV-04-00072.pdf.

87 James Thorp, MD, "Miscarriage of Science," *The Highwire*, Episode 293, Nov. 10, 2022, thehighwire.com/videos/episode-293-miscarriage-of-science.

88 James A. Thorp et al., "COVID-19 Vaccines: The Impact on Pregnancy Outcomes and Menstrual Function," *Preprints* (2022): 2022090430, doi: 10.20944/preprints202209.0430.v1.

89 @LeilaniDowding, "Kimberly Bliss MD, Confirms a 50% Decrease in Fertility Rate and a 50% Increase in Miscarriage Rate 25% increase in Pap smears and cervical malignancies," Twitter, Oct 17, 2022, twitter.com/LeilaniDowding/status/1582011477606936576.

90 "Neonatal Deaths Review Announced," Scottish Government, Sep. 30, 2022, gov.scot/news/neonatal-deaths-review-announced.

91 "Investigation into Spike in Newborn Baby Deaths in Scotland," BBC, Nov. 19, 2021, bbc.com/news/uk-scotland-59347464.

92 "VAERS COVID Vaccine Reproductive Health Related Reports," OpenVAERS, through Jan. 27, 2023, openvaers.com/covid-data/reproductive-health.

93 Mason Johnson, "How to Select a Midwife: Questions to Ask a Midwife?", Choices in Childbirth, Sep. 9, 2021, web.archive.org/web/20230206035148/https://en.choicesinchildbirth.org/how-to-select-a-midwife/.

94 David A. Anderson and Gabrielle M. Gilkison, "The Cost of Home Birth in the United States," *International Journal of Environmental Research and Public Health* 18, no. 19 (2021): 10361, doi: 10.3390/ijerph181910361.

95 Henci Goer, "Dueling Statistics: Is Out-of-Hospital Birth Safe?" *Journal of Perinatal Education* 25, no. 2 (2016): 75–79, doi: 10.1891/1058-1243.25.2.75.

96 Meredith Deliso, "How COVID-19 Continues to Impact Birthing Practices," ABC, Mar. 5, 2022, abcnews.go.com/Health/covid-19-continues-impact-birthing-practices/story?id=83046601.

97 Teresa Janevic et al., "Pandemic Birthing: Childbirth Satisfaction, Perceived Health Care Bias, and Postpartum Health During the COVID-19 Pandemic," *Maternal and Child Health Journal* 25, no. 6 (2021): 860–869, doi: 10.1007/s10995-021-03158-8.

98 "Consumers Estimate your Healthcare Expenses," Fair Health Consumer, accessed Aug. 1, 2023, fairhealthconsumer.org.

99 Renee Y Hsia, Yaa Akosa Antwi, and Ellerie Weber, "Analysis of Variation in Charges and Prices Paid for Vaginal and Caesarean Section Births: A Cross-Sectional Study," *BMJ Open* 4, no. 1 (2014): e004017, doi: 10.1136/bmjopen-2013-004017.

100 "Having a Doula – What Are the Benefits?", American Pregnancy Association, accessed Dec. 30, 2022, americanpregnancy.org/healthy

-pregnancy/labor-and-birth/having-a-doula.

101 "Planned Home Birth," American College of Obstetricians and Gynecologists, no. 697 (2017), acog.org/clinical/clinical-guidance/committee-opinion/articles/2017/04/planned-home-birth.

102 "More Women Choosing Home Births Since Pandemic: 'You Have a Lot More Freedom.'" *The Defender*, Nov. 10, 2021, childrenshealthdefense.org/defender/chd-tv-tea-time-polly-tommey-sheelee-rock-doula-home-births-covid.

103 "Lamaze Healthy Birth Practices," Lamaze, accessed Dec. 30, 2022, lamaze.org/childbirth-practices.

104 "What Are the Options for Pain Relief During Labor and Delivery?", National Institute of Child Health and Human Development, accessed Dec. 30, 2022, nichd.nih.gov/health/topics/labor-delivery/topicinfo/pain-relief.

105 Jill Cohen, "The Homebirth Choice," *Midwifery Today*, updated September 2008, midwiferytoday.com/web-article/the-homebirth-choice.

106 Anderson and Gilkison, 2021.

107 American Association of Birth Centers | AABC, accessed Aug. 1, 2023, birthcenters.org.

108 Aviva Romm, "Why We Need Birthing Centers," On Health: A Podcast for Women, accessed Feb. 13, 2023, avivaromm.com/birthing-centers.

109 "Psychoprophylaxis," The Free Dictionary, accessed Dec. 30, 2022, thefreedictionary.com/psychoprophylaxis.

110 Lamaze International, accessed Aug. 1, 2023, lamaze.org.

111 Anthony Lathrop, Carrie F. Bonsack, and David M. Haas, "Women's Experiences with Water Birth: A Matched Groups Prospective Study," *Birth* 45, no. 4 (2018): 416–423, doi: 10.1111/birt.12362.

112 International Childbirth Education Association, "Water Labor & Water Birth," ICEA Position Paper, October 2015, icea.org/wp-content/uploads/2016/01/Water_Birth_PP.pdf.

113 "The Complete Guide to the Alexander Technique," Alexander Technique, accessed Aug. 1, 2023, alexandertechnique.com.

114 "The Bradley Method," Bradley Birth, accessed Aug. 1, 2023, bradleybirth.com.

115 Ivan Hand, Lawrence Noble, and Steven A. Abrams, "Vitamin K and the Newborn Infant," *Pediatrics* 149, no. 3 (2022): e2021056036, doi: 10.1542/peds.2021-056036.

116 "What Is Vitamin K Deficiency Bleeding?" Centers for Disease Control and Prevention, last reviewed Feb. 10, 2023, cdc.gov/ncbddd/vitamink/facts.html.

117 "Vitamin K Shots," Children's Health Defense, Feb. 13, 2020, childrenshealthdefense.org/protecting-our-future/vitamin-k-shots.

118 VITAMIN K1 INJECTION, Pfizer, labeling.pfizer.com/ShowLabeling.aspx?id=5392.

119 "Vitamin K1 Prescribing Information," Drugs.com, updated Aug. 22, 2022, drugs.com/pro/vitamin-k1.html.

120 Jaspreet Loyal and Eugene D. Shapiro, "Refusal of Intramuscular Vitamin K by Parents of Newborns: A Review," *Hospital Pediatrics* 10, no. 3 (2020): 286–294, doi: 10.1542/hpeds.2019-0228.

121 Sam McCulloch, "Vitamin K Shot for Baby at Birth," BellyBelly, Apr. 28, 2021 (updated Dec. 6, 2022), bellybelly.com.au/baby/vitamin-k-shot.

122 "Hepatitis B Virus: A Comprehensive Strategy for Eliminating Transmission in the United States Through Universal Childhood Vaccination. Recommendations of the Immunization Practices Advisory Committee (ACIP)," *Morbidity and Mortality Weekly Report* 40, no. RR-13 (1991): 1–19, PMID: 1835756, bit.ly/43PBu8L.

123 Centers for Disease Control Epidemiology Program Office, "Summary of Notifiable Diseases, United States, 1990," *Morbidity and Mortality Weekly Report* 39, no. 53 (1991), PMID: 1656184, stacks.cdc.gov/view/cdc/35905.

124 Mary S. Holland, "Compulsory Vaccination, the Constitution, and the Hepatitis B Mandate for Infants and Young Children," *Yale Journal of Health Policy, Law, and Ethics* 12, no. 1 (2012): 39, papers.ssrn.com/sol3/papers.cfm?abstract_id=2039392.

125 David A. Geier et al., "A Longitudinal Cohort Study of the Relationship Between Thimerosal-Containing Hepatitis B Vaccination and Specific Delays in Development in the United States: Assessment of Attributable Risk and Lifetime Care Costs," *Journal of Epidemiology and Global Health* 6, no. 2 (2016): 105–118, doi: 10.1016/j.jegh.2015.06.002.

126 "Merck's Recombivax Vaccine Shortage Causes Reduced Deaths in Babies—A Natural Experiment?", Children's Health Defense, Jan. 22, 2019, childrenshealthdefense.org/news/mercks-recombivax-vaccine-shortage-causes-reduced-deaths-in-babies-a-natural-experiment.

127 Heidi Stevenson, "Yeast in Vaccines Tied to Autoimmune Diseases," Children's Health Defense, Mar. 27, 2018, childrenshealthdefense.org/news/yeast-in-vaccines-tied-to-autoimmune-diseases.

128 "The Changing Face of Vaccinology," Children's Health Defense, Apr. 3, 2018, childrenshealthdefense.org/news/the-changing-face-of-vaccinology.

129 JB Handley, "Vax-Unvax Study of Mice Implicates Hepatitis B Vaccine—Media Silent," Children's Health Defense, May 17, 2018, childrenshealthdefense.org/news/vax-unvax-study-of-mice-implicates-hepatitis-b-vaccine-media-silent.

130 JB Handley, "New Study: Hep B Vaccine 'May Have Adverse Implications for Brain Development and Cognition,'" Children's Health Defense, Jul. 26, 2018, childrenshealthdefense.org/news/new-study-hep-b-vaccine-may-have-adverse-implications-for-brain-development-and-cognition.

131 Engerix-B, accessed Aug. 1, 2023, fda.gov/media/119403/download.

132 Recombivax HB, accessed Aug. 1, 2023, bit.ly/3qb6B.

133 Thomson et al., 1995.

134 Elizabeth R. Moore et al., "Early Skin-to-Skin Contact for Mothers and Their Healthy Newborn Infants," *Cochrane Database of Systematic Reviews* 11, no. 11 (2016): CD003519, doi: 10.1002/14651858.CD003519.pub4.

135 Efrem S. Lim et al., "Early Life Dynamics of the Human Gut Virome and Bacterial Microbiome in Infants," *Nature Medicine* 21, no. 10 (2015): 1228–1234, doi: 10.1038/nm.3950.

136 Irene Yang et al., "The Infant Microbiome: Implications for Infant Health and Neurocognitive Development," *Nursing Research* 65, no. 1 (2016): 76–88, doi: 10.1097/NNR.0000000000000133.

137 Benedetta Raspini et al., "Prenatal and Postnatal Determinants in Shaping Offspring's Microbiome in the First 1000 Days: Study Protocol and Preliminary Results at 1 Month of Life," *Italian Journal of Pediatrics* 46

(2020): 45, doi: 10.1186/s13052-020 -0794-8.

138 Ruairi C. Robertson et al., "The Human Microbiome and Child Growth — First 1000 Days and Beyond," *Trends in Microbiology* 27, no. 2 (2019): 131–147, doi: 10.1016/j .tim.2018.09.008.

139 Robertson et al., 2019.

140 "Breastfeeding." Centers for Disease Control and Prevention, accessed Jan. 4, 2023, cdc.gov/breastfeeding /data/facts.html.

141 D.A. Sela et al., "The Genome Sequence of *Bifidobacterium longum* subsp. *infantis* Reveals Adaptations for Milk Utilization Within the Infant Microbiome," *Proceedings of the National Academy of Sciences of the United States of America* 105, no. 48 (2008): 18964–18969, doi: 10.1073 /pnas.0809584105.

142 Kelsey Fehr et al., "Breastmilk Feeding Practices Are Associated with the Co-Occurrence of Bacteria in Mothers' Milk and the Infant Gut: the CHILD Cohort Study," *Cell Host & Microbe* 28, no. 2 (2020): 285–297. e4, doi: 10.1016/j.chom.2020.06.009.

143 Shirin Moossavi et al., "Composition and Variation of the Human Milk Microbiota Are Influenced by Maternal and Early-Life Factors," *Cell Host & Microbe* 25, no. 2 (2019): 324–335 .e4, doi: 10.1016/j.chom.2019.01.011.

144 Jen Allbritton, "Nourishing a Growing Baby," Weston A. Price Foundation, Oct. 19, 2005, westonaprice.org/health-topics /childrens-health/nourishing-a -growing-baby.

145 Robert S. Mendelsohn, *How to Raise a Healthy Child... in Spite of Your Doctor*, Ballantine Books, 1987.

146 Patricia Palmeira and Magda Carneiro-Sampaio, "Immunology of Breast Milk," *Revista da Associação Médica Brasileira* 62, no. 6 (2016): 584–593, doi: 10.1590/1806-9282 .62.06.584.

147 Thaidra Gaufin, Nicole H. Tobin, and Grace M. Aldrovandi, "The Importance of the Microbiome in Pediatrics and Pediatric Infectious Diseases," *Current Opinion in Pediatrics* 30, no. 1 (2018): 117–124, doi: 10.1097 /MOP.0000000000000576.

148 Colin Binns, MiKyung Lee, and Wah Yun Low, "The Long-Term Public Health Benefits of Breastfeeding," *Asia-Pacific Journal of Public Health* 28, no. 1 (2016): 7–14, doi: 10.1177/10105 39515624964.

149 Eyal Klement et al., "Breastfeeding and Risk of Inflammatory Bowel Disease: A Systematic Review with Meta-Analysis," *American Journal of Clinical Nutrition* 80, no. 5 (2004): 1342–1352, doi: 10.1093 /ajcn/80.5.1342.

150 Camilla Henriksson, Anee-Marie Boström, and Ingela E. Wiklund, "What Effect Does Breastfeeding Have on Coeliac Disease? A Systematic Review Update," *Evidence-Based Medicine* 18, no. 3 (2013): 98–103, doi: 10.1136 /eb-2012-100607.

151 Vânia Vieira Borba, Kassem Sharif, and Yehuda Shoenfeld, "Breastfeeding and Autoimmunity: Programing Health from the Beginning," *American Journal of Reproductive Immunology* 79, no. 1 (2018), doi: 10.1111/aji.12778.

152 U.K. Childhood Cancer Study Investigators, "Breastfeeding and Childhood Cancer," *British Journal of Cancer* 85, no. 11 (2001): 1685–1694, doi: 10.1054/bjoc.2001.2110.

153 Brian S. Hooker and Neil Z. Miller, "Health Effects in Vaccinated Versus Unvaccinated Children, with Covariates for Breastfeeding Status and Type of Birth," *Journal of Translational Science* 7 (2021): 1–11, doi: 10.15761/JTS.1000459.

154 Kathleen Lange et al., "Effects of Antibiotics on Gut Microbiota," *Digestive Diseases* 34, no. 3 (2016): 260–268, doi: 10.1159/000443360.

155 Natasha Campbell-McBride, "Gut and Psychology Syndrome (GAPS)," Weston A. Price Foundation, Mar. 22, 2009, westonaprice.org/health -topics/childrens-health/gut-and -psychology-syndrome-gaps.

156 Nicole D. White, "Drug-Induced Microbiome Changes: Considerations in Pregnancy," *American Journal of Lifestyle Medicine* 17, no. 1 (2022): 50–53, doi: 10.1177/15598276221130259.

157 Mara J. Dinsmoor et al., "Use of Intrapartum Antibiotics and the Incidence of Postnatal Maternal and Neonatal Yeast Infections," *Obstetrics and Gynecology* 106, no. 1 (2005): 19–22, doi: 10.1097/01 .AOG.0000164049.12159.bd.

158 Eileen K. Hutton et al., "Associations of Intrapartum Antibiotics and Growth, Atopy, Gastrointestinal and Sleep Outcomes at One Year of Age," *Pediatric Research* (2023 Feb 18), doi: 10.1038/s41390-023-02525-1.

159 Olli Turta and Samuli Rautava, "Antibiotics, Obesity and the Link to Microbes – What Are We Doing to Our Children?", *BMC Medicine* 14 (2016): 57, doi: 10.1186/s12916-016 -0605-7.

160 Qiuji Tao et al., "Prenatal Exposure to Antibiotics and Risk of Neurodevelopmental Disorders in Offspring: A Systematic Review and Meta-Analysis," *Frontiers in Neurology* 13 (2022): 1045865, doi: 10.3389/fneur.2022.1045865.

161 P. Brandon Bookstaver et al., "A Review of Antibiotic Use in Pregnancy," *Pharmacotherapy* 35, no. 11 (2015): 1052–1062, doi: 10.1002 /phar.1649.

162 Christa Novelli, "Treating Group B Strep: Are Antibiotics Necessary?", *Mothering Magazine*, Issue 121, Nov/ Dec 2003, birthspirit.com/wp -content/uploads/2014/03/GBS -Mothering-article.pdf.

163 Children's Health Defense Team, "Prenatal Care, American Style—A Trojan Horse for Harmful Interventions?", *The Defender*, Sep. 29, 2022, childrenshealthdefense.org /defender/prenatal-infant-maternal -mortality-harmful-interventions/.

164 Lindsey VanAlstyne, "Natural Remedies for Group B Strep in Pregnancy," *Mother Rising*, updated Sep. 3, 2022, motherrisingbirth.com /2016/09/natural-remedies-for-group -b-strep.html.

165 Fiona M. Smaill and Rosalie M. Grivell, "Antibiotic Prophylaxis Versus No Prophylaxis for Preventing Infection After Cesarean Section," *The Cochrane Database of Systematic Reviews* 2014, no. 10 (2014): CD007482, doi: 10.1002/14651858.CD007482.pub3.

166 Kristin Lawless, "The Bacteria Babies Need," originally published in the *New York Times*, Jun. 17, 2018, kristinlawless.com/news/2018/6/22 /the-bacteria-babies-need.

167 Maciej Chichlowski et al., "*Bifidobacterium longum* Subspecies *infantis* (B. infantis) in Pediatric Nutrition: Current State of Knowledge," *Nutrients* 12, no. 6 (2020): 1581, doi: 10.3390/nu12061 581.

168 Claire E. O'Brien et al., "Early Probiotic Supplementation with B. infantis in Breastfed Infants Leads to Persis1ot Colonization at 1 Year," *Pediatric Research* 91, no. 3 (2022): 627–636, doi: 10.1038/s41390-020 -01350-0.

169 Natasha K. Sriraman and Ann Kellams, "Breastfeeding: What Are the Barriers? Why Women Struggle to Achieve Their Goals," *Journal of Women's Health* 25, no. 7 (2016):

714–722, doi: 10.1089/jwh .2014.5059.

170 "USLCA's Find An IBCLC® Directory," United States Lactation Consultant Association, accessed Aug. 1, 2023, uslca.org/resources /find-an-ibclc.

171 "Find A Doula," Doula International, accessed Aug. 1, 2023, dona.org /what-is-a-doula/find-a-doula.

172 "How to Treat and Prevent Mastitis," American Pregnancy Association, accessed Dec. 31, 2022, americanpregnancy.org/healthy -pregnancy/breastfeeding/how-to -treat-and-prevent-mastitis/.

173 "Mastitis," La Leche League International, accessed Dec. 31, 2022, llli.org/breastfeeding-info /mastitis/.

174 Karen Cuni, "Exclusive Pumping," Breastfeeding USA, 2014, breast feedingusa.org/content/article /exclusive-pumping.

175 Human Milk Banking, accessed, Aug. 1, 2023, hmbana.org.

176 "Homemade Baby Formula," Weston A. Price Foundation, Dec. 31, 2001, westonaprice.org/health-topics /childrens-health/formula -homemade-baby-formula.

177 Kaayla Daniel, "The Brilliance and Courage of Dr. Mary Enig," Weston A. Price Foundation, Sep. 10, 2014, westonaprice.org/health-topics/soy -alert/the-brilliance-and-courage -of-dr-mary-enig.

178 "Baby Formula Shortage Solutions with Founding President, Weston A. Price Foundation," CHD.TV, May 20, 2022, live.childrenshealthdefense.org /chd-tv/shows/good-morning-chd /baby-formula-shortage-solutions -with-founding-president-weston -a-price-foundation/.

179 "Search Results for "Infant Formula," *Drug Watch*, accessed Aug. 1, 2023, drugwatch.com /search/?query=infant+formula.

180 Jake Johnson, "Abbott Issued $5 Billion in Stock Buybacks While Tainted Formula Sickened Babies," *The Defender*, May 23, 2022, childrenshealthdefense.org /defender/abbott-stock-buybacks -tainted-formula-sickened-babies.

181 "Looking for European Baby Formula? Many American Parents Are," *Daily Sundial*, May 27, 2021, sundial.csun.edu/164839 /sundialbrandstudio/sundial -marketplace/looking-for -european-baby-formula-many -american-parents-are.

182 Niamh Michail, "Improving Infant Formula with Synthetic Biology," *Fi Global Insights*, Feb. 13, 2023, insights.figlobal.com/new-product -development/improving-infant -formula-synthetic-biology.

183 Bridget Young, "Your Ultimate Guide to Choosing the Best Organic Formula," Baby Formula Expert, Nov. 14, 2020, web.archive.org/web /20230321111005/https://babyformula expert.com/guide-to-organic -formula/.

184 A. Leung and A. Otley, "Concerns for the Use of Soy-based Formulas in Infant Nutrition," *Paediatrics & Child Health* 14, no. 2 (2009): 109–113, doi: 10.1093/pch/14.2.109.

185 Merinda Teller, "Soy Infant Formula and Autism," Weston A. Price Foundation, Oct. 27, 2016, westonaprice.org/health-topics /childrens-health/soy-infant -formula-autism.

186 "The Tragedy of Soy Infant Formula," Weston A. Price Foundation, Jan. 1, 2000, westonaprice.org/health-topics/soy -alert/the-tragedy-of-soy-infant -formula.

187 "Action Is Needed Now to Lower the Content of Aluminum in Infant Formulas," *ScienceDaily*, Oct. 10, 2013, sciencedaily.com/releases/2013 /10/131010091429.htm.

188 Jillian Levy, "Acid Reflux Diet: Best Foods, Foods to Avoid & Supplements that Help," Dr. Axe, Feb. 28, 2017, draxe.com/health /acid-reflux-diet/.

189 Steven J. Czinn and Samra Blanchard, "Gastroesophageal Reflux Disease in Neonates and Infants: When and How to Treat," *Paediatric Drugs* 15, no. 1 (2013): 19–27, doi.org /10.1007/s40272-012-0004-2.

190 Trish Ringley, "Reflux in Preemies," VeryWellHealth, updated Feb. 17, 2023, verywellhealth.com/reflux-in -preemies-2748637.

191 Kathryne Pirtle, "Acid Reflux: A Red Flag," Weston A. Price Foundation, Jun. 25, 2010, westonaprice.org /health-topics/modern-diseases /acid-reflux-a-red-flag.

192 Jen Allbritton, "Calming the Cry of Colic," Weston A. Price Foundation, Aug. 24, 2006, westonaprice.org /health-topics/childrens-health /calming-the-cry-of-colic.

193 Ringley, 2022.

194 Mark Safe et al., "Widespread Use of Gastric Acid Inhibitors in Infants: Are They Needed? Are They Safe?", *World Journal of Gastrointestinal Pharmacology and Therapeutics* 7, no. 4 (2016): 531–539, doi: 10.4292 /wjgpt.v7.i4.531.

195 "The Method," Svetlana Masgutova Educational Institute, accessed Mar. 18, 2023, masgutovamethod.com /the-method.

196 Min Sohn, Youngmee Ahn, and Sangmi Lee, "Assessment of Primitive Reflexes in High-risk Newborns," *Journal of Clinical Medicine Research* 3, no. 6 (2011): 285–290, doi: 10.4021/jocmr706w.

197 Taylor Norris, "Is My Newborn's Heavy Breathing Typical?", Healthline, Jul. 15, 2022, healthline. com/health/newborn-breathing #normal-breathing.

198 Tahiat Mahboob, "How We Breathe Has Major Impacts on Our Body— James Nestor Has Recommendations to Improve It," CBC Radio, Jul. 25, 2021, cbc.ca/radio/sunday/the -sunday-magazine-for-january-17 -2021-1.5874646/how-we-breathe -has-major-impacts-on-our-body -james-nestor-has-recommendations -to-improve-it-1.5874681.

199 K. Kairaitis et al., "Route of Breathing in Patients with Asthma," *Chest* 116, no. 6 (1999): 1646–1652, doi: 10.1378/chest.116.6.1646.

200 Mervat Hallani, John R. Wheatley, and Terence C. Amis, "Enforced Mouth Breathing Decreases Lung Function in Mild Asthmatics," *Respirology* 13, no. 4 (2008): 553–558, doi: 10.1111/j.1440-1843 .2008.01300.x.

201 Ju-Yeon Jung and Chang-Ki Kang, "Investigation on the Effect of Oral Breathing on Cognitive Activity Using Functional Brain Imaging," *Healthcare (Basel)* 9, no. 6 (2021): 645, doi: 10.3390/healthcare9060645.

202 "Signs of Respiratory Distress in Your Infant," Seattle Children's Hospital Research Foundation, Revised 8/22 PE1736, accessed Aug. 1, 2023, seattlechildrens.org/pdf /PE1736.pdf.

203 Pauline F.F. Decima et al., "The Longitudinal Effects of Persis10t Periodic Breathing on Cerebral Oxygenation in Preterm Infants," *Sleep Medicine* 16, no. 6 (2015): 729– 735, doi: 10.1016/j.sleep.2015.02.537.

204 Dorothy H. Kelly and Daniel C. Shannon, "Periodic Breathing in Infants with Near-Miss Sudden Infant Death Syndrome," Pediatrics 63, no. 3 (1979): 355–360, PMID: 440836.

205 Viera Scheibner, "The Real Cause of Cot Death (SIDS)," *Health Impact News*, Feb. 19, 2018, vaccineimpact.com

/2018/what-are-the-real-causes-of-sudden-infant-death-syndrome-sids-why-are-vaccines-excluded.

206 Neil Z. Miller, "Vaccines and Sudden Infant Death: An Analysis of the VAERS database 1990–2019 and Review of the Medical Literature," *Toxicology Reports* 8 (2021): 1324–1335, doi: 10.1016/j.toxrep.2021.06.020.

207 Yuh-Jyh Lin et al., "Periodic Breathing in Term Infants – Is It Benign? 950," *Pediatric Research* 41, suppl 4 (1997): 161, doi.org/10.1203/00006450-199704001-00969.

208 "Newborn Sleep: A Discussion with Elizabeth Pantley," KellyMom, Jan. 15, 2018, kellymom.com/parenting/nighttime/newborn-sleep-a-discussion-with-elizabeth-pantley.

209 Centers for Disease Control and Prevention, "Safe Sleep for Babies," Vital Signs, updated Nov. 27, 2018, web.archive.org/web/20230112110046/https://www.cdc.gov/vitalsigns/safesleep/index.html.

210 William G. Gilroy, "Researchers Propose 'Breastsleeping' as a New Word and Concept," Notre Dame News, Sep. 24, 2015, news.nd.edu/news/researchers-propose-breastsleeping-as-a-new-word-and-concept.

211 "Does Nighttime Breastfeeding Cause Cavities?" Ask Dr. Sears, accessed Mar. 18, 2023, askdrsears.com/topics/feeding-eating/breastfeeding/faqs/breastfeeding-and-cavities.

212 Kelly Bonyata, "Is Breastfeeding Linked to Tooth Decay?" KellyMom, Mar. 27, 2018, kellymom.com/ages/older-infant/tooth-decay.

213 Jessica, "Nighttime Breastfeeding Does Not Cause Cavities," Cure Tooth Decay, accessed Mar. 18, 2023, curetoothdecay.com/blog/nighttime-breastfeeding-does-not-cause-cavities.

214 Centers for Disease Control and Prevention, "Safe Sleep for Babies," 2018, web.archive.org/web/20200612103850/https://www.cdc.gov/vitalsigns/safesleep/index.html.

215 James J. McKenna and Thomas McDade, "Why Babies Should Never Sleep Alone: a Review of the Co-sleeping Controversy in Relation to SIDS, Bedsharing and Breast Feeding," *Paediatric Respiratory Reviews* 6, no. 2 (2005):134–152, doi: 10.1016/j.prrv.2005.03.006.

216 Gilroy, 2015.

217 Arianna Huffington, "My Conversation with Co-Sleeping Expert James McKenna," *HuffPost*, updated Dec. 4, 2015, huffpost.com/entry/james-mckenna-co-sleeping-expert_b_7119782.

218 Yi Huang et al., "Influence of Bedsharing Activity on Breastfeeding Duration Among US Mothers," *JAMA Pediatrics* 167, no. 11 (2013): 1038–1044, doi: 10.1001/jamapediatrics.2013.2632.

219 Megan Trimble, "U.S. Kids More Likely to Die Than Kids in 19 Other Nations," *U.S. News*, Jan. 11, 2018, usnews.com/news/best-countries/articles/2018-01-11/us-has-highest-child-mortality-rate-of-20-rich-countries.

220 Neil Z. Miller and Gary S. Goldman, "Infant Mortality Rates Regressed Against Number of Vaccine Doses Routinely Given: Is There a Biochemical or Synergistic Toxicity?", *Human & Experimental Toxicology* 30, no. 9 (2011): 1420–1428, doi: 10.1177/0960327111407644.

221 Gary S. Goldman and Neil Z. Miller, "Reaffirming a Positive Correlation Between Number of Vaccine Doses and Infant Mortality Rates: A Response to Critics," Cureus 15, no. 2 (2023): e34566, doi: 10.7759/cureus.34566.

222 Michael Nevradakis, "Higher Infant Mortality Rates Linked to Higher Number of Vaccine Doses, New Study Confirms," *The Defender*, Feb. 7, 2023, childrenshealthdefense.org/defender/infant-mortality-vaccine-doses.

223 Angela Morrow, "The 10 Leading Causes of Infant Death," *Verywell Health*, Nov. 15, 2021, verywellhealth.com/leading-causes-of-infant-death-1132374.

224 "Sudden Unexpected Infant Death and Sudden Infant Death Syndrome: Data and Statistics," Centers for Disease Control and Prevention, reviewed Jun. 21, 2022, cdc.gov/sids/data.htm.

225 Brian Hooker, "58% of Infant Deaths Reported to VAERS Occurred Within 3 Days of Vaccination, Research Shows," *The Defender*, Aug. 3, 2021, childrenshealthdefense.org/defender/right-on-point-wayne-rohde-neil-miller-infant-deaths-reported-vaers-vaccination.

226 "Inventing Diagnoses to Cover Up Vaccine Injury—a Con as Old as Vaccination Itself," *The Defender*, Jul. 27, 2022, childrenshealthdefense.org/defender/vaccine-injury-cover-up-covid-vaccination.

227 Alan R. Hinman, Walter A. Orenstein, and Anne Schuchat, "Vaccine-Preventable Diseases, Immunizations, and MMWR—1961–2011," *MMWR Supplements* 60, no. 4 (2011): 49–57, bit.ly/44NYsyt.

228 "Recommended Vaccinations for Infants and Children, Parent-Friendly Version," Centers for Disease Control and Prevention, reviewed Feb. 10, 2023, cdc.gov/vaccines/schedules/easy-to-read/child-easyread.html.

229 "Sudden Infant Death Syndrome," *Encyclopedia.com*, updated May 29, 2018, encyclopedia.com/medicine/diseases-and-conditions/pathology/sudden-infant-death-syndrome.

230 Miller, 2021.

231 Stefano D'Errico et al., "Beta-tryptase and Quantitative Mast-Cell Increase in a Sudden Infant Death Following Hexavalent Immunization," *Forensic Science International* 179, no. 2–3 (2008): e25–e29, doi: 10.1016/j.forsciint.2008.04.018.

232 L. Matturri, G. Del Corno, and A.M. Lavezzi, "Sudden Infant Death Following Hexavalent Vaccination: a Neuropathologic Study," *Current Medicinal Chemistry* 21, no. 7 (2014): 941–946, doi: 10.2174/09298673113206660289.

233 "CDC, FDA Prepare Mass Distribution of a Merck/Sanofi 6-in-One Vaccine for Kids, Turning Blind Eye to Safety Signals," *The Defender*, Jun. 25, 2021, childrenshealthdefense.org/defender/cdc-fda-vaxelis-vaccine-merck-sanofi-kids.

234 Lyn Redwood, "Court Hears Gardasil Science and Moves Forward," Children's Health Defense, Jan. 29, 2019, childrenshealthdefense.org/news/court-hears-gardasil-science-and-moves-forward.

235 Brian Hooker, "During COVID Lockdown, Vaccine Rates Dropped—So Did the Number of SIDS Deaths," *The Defender*, Jan. 22, 2021, childrenshealthdefense.org/defender/covid-lockdown-vaccine-rates-dropped-so-did-sids-deaths.

236 "A COVID Silver Lining? More Parents Than Ever Questioning 'Routine' Childhood Vaccines," *The Defender*, Aug. 12, 2022, childrenshealthdefense.org/defender/parents-questioning-routine-childhood-vaccines-covid.

237 Brian S. Hooker and Neil Z. Miller, "Analysis of Health Outcomes in Vaccinated and Unvaccinated Children: Developmental Delays, Asthma, Ear Infections and Gastrointestinal Disorders," *SAGE*

Open Medicine 8 (2020), doi.org /10.1177/2050312120925344.

238 Anthony R. Mawson et al., "Pilot Comparative Study on the Health of Vaccinated and Unvaccinated 6- to 12-year-old U.S. Children," *Journal of Translational Science* 3, no. 3 (2017): 1–12, doi: 10.15761/JTS.1000186.

239 Alix Mayer, "Groundbreaking Study Shows Unvaccinated Children Are Healthier Than Vaccinated Children," *The Defender*, Dec. 7, 2020, childrenshealthdefense.org /defender/unvaccinated-children -healthier-than-vaccinated-children.

240 Manda Aufochs Gillespie, "Baby Care Products Expose Infants to Toxic Chemicals," EcoParent, Aug. 16, 2019, ecoparent.ca/eco-wellness /baby-care-products-expose -infants-toxic-chemicals.

241 S. Behring, "Helpful Tips for Diaper Rash: What You Need to Know," Healthline, updated Feb, 2023, healthline.com/health/home -remedies-diaper-rash#risk-factors.

242 "Natural Cures for Diaper Rash," Earth Clinic, modified Sep. 22, 2017, earthclinic.com/children/diaper-rash .html.

243 Megan Redshaw, "J&J Eyes Bankruptcy Maneuver in Bid to Skirt Liability in Baby Powder Lawsuits," *The Defender*, Jul. 19, 2021, childrenshealthdefense.org /defender/johnson-johnson -bankruptcy-liability-baby-powder -lawsuits.

244 Jen Allbritton, "Cloth Diapers Made Simple...Promise!" Weston A. Price Foundation, Jul. 16, 2006, westonaprice.org/health-topics /childrens-health/cloth-diapers -made-simple-promise.

245 Sydney Swanson and Nneka Lieba, "EWG's Healthy Living: Quick Tips to Safer Diapers," Environmental Working Group, Dec. 10, 2020, ewg.org /research/diaper-guide.

246 John Moody, "Raising Baby with Safer—and Less—Stuff," Weston A. Price Foundation, Apr. 28, 2021, westonaprice.org/health-topics /raising-baby-with-safer-and-less -stuff.

247 Motherly, accessed Aug. 1, 2023, mother.ly.

248 Alexandre Faisal-Cury et al., "The Impact of Postpartum Depression and Bonding Impairment on Child Development at 12 to 15 Months After Delivery," *Journal of Affective Disorders Reports* 4 (2021): 100125, doi.org/10.1016/j.jadr.2021.100125.

249 "Depression in Pregnant Women and Mothers: How Children Are Affected," *Paediatrics Child Health* 9, no. 8 (2004): 584–586, doi: 10.1093 /pch/9.8.584.

250 Postpartum Support International, accessed Aug. 1, 2023, postpartum .net/learn-more.

251 Crystal Edler Schiller, Samantha Meltzer-Brody, and David R. Rubinow, "The Role of Reproductive Hormones in Postpartum Depression," *CNS Spectrums* 20, no. 1 (2015): 48–59, doi: 10.1017/S1092 852914000480.

252 Jolene Brighten, "Postpartum Thyroiditis," Dr. Jolene Brighten, Mar. 8, 2015, drbrighten.com /postpartum-thyroiditis.

253 Ellen C.G. Grant, "Zinc and Copper Deficiencies Can Cause Postpartum Depression," Rapid Response to Roshni R. Patel, Deirdre J. Murphy, and Tim J. Peters, "Operative Delivery and Postnatal Depression: A Cohort Study," *The BMJ* 330 (2005): 879, doi: 10.1136/bmj.38376.603426 .D3.

254 Simone Hagmeyer, Jasmin Carmen Haderspeck, and Andreas Martin Grabrucker, "Behavioral Impairments in Animal Models for Zinc Deficiency," *Frontiers in Behavioral Neuroscience* 8 (2015): 443, doi.org/10.3389/fnbeh.2014.00443.

255 Grant, 2005.

256 "PSI Online Support Meetings," Postpartum Support International, accessed Aug. 1, 2023, postpartum .net/get-help/psi-online-support -meetings.

257 Joy Anderson, Kathryn Malley, and Robynne Snell, "Is 6 Months Still the Best for Exclusive Breastfeeding and Introduction of Solids? A Literature Review with Consideration to the Risk of the Development of Allergies," *Breastfeeding Review* 17, no. 2 (2009): 23–31, PMID: 19685855.

258 Sally Fallon Morell, "Bringing Up Baby: When to Wean ... and How," Weston A. Price Foundation, Apr. 26, 2021, westonaprice.org/health -topics/bringing-up-baby-when-to -weanand-how.

259 Dr. Alan Greene and Anna Lappé, "Why Organic Is the Right Choice for Parents," *TIME*, Jun. 23, 2014, time. com/2914155/organic-food -children-health.

260 Amanda Macmillan and Julia Naftulin, "4 Science-Backed Health Benefits of Eating Organic," *TIME*, Jul. 27, 2017, time.com/4871915 /health-benefits-organic-food.

261 Lynn Razaitis, "The Liver Files," Weston A. Price Foundation, Jul. 29, 2005, westonaprice.org/health -topics/food-features/the-liver-files.

262 "Children's Health," Weston A. Price Foundation, accessed Feb. 16, 2023, westonaprice.org/childrens-health.

263 Allbritton, "Nourishing a Growing Baby," 2005.

264 Ruchi S. Gupta et al., "The Prevalence, Severity, and Distribution of Childhood Food Allergy in the United States," *Pediatrics* 128, no. 1 (2011): e9–e17, doi: 10.1542/peds.2011-0204.

265 Kris10 D. Jackson, Lajeana D. Howie, and Lara J. Akinbami, "Trends in Allergic Conditions Among Children: United States, 1997–2011," Centers for Disease Control and Prevention, NCHS Data Brief, no. 121 (May 2013), cdc.gov/nchs/products/databriefs /db121.htm.

266 Megan S. Motosue et al., "National Trends in Emergency Department Visits and Hospitalizations for Food-Induced Anaphylaxis in US Children," *Pediatric Allergy and Immunology* 29, no. 5 (2018): 538–544, doi: 10.1111/pai.12908.

267 "Claim Lines with Diagnoses of Anaphylactic Food Reactions Climbed 377 Percent from 2007 to 2016," FAIR Health, Aug. 22, 2017, fairhealth.org/press-release /claim-lines-with-diagnoses -of-anaphylactic-food-reactions -climbed-377-percent-from-2007 -to-2016.

268 "Vaccine Excipient Summary," Centers for Disease Control and Prevention, Nov. 1, 2021, cdc.gov /vaccines/pubs/pinkbook/downloads /appendices/b/excipient-table-2.pdf.

269 Vinu Arumugham, "Evidence that Food Proteins in Vaccines Cause the Development of Food Allergies and Its Implications for Vaccine Policy," *Journal of Developing Drugs* 4, no. 4 (2015): 137, doi: 10.4172/2329 -6631.1000137.

270 Todd D. Terhune and Richard C. Deth, "A Role for Impaired Regulatory T Cell Function in Adverse Responses to Aluminum Adjuvant-Containing Vaccines in Genetically Susceptible Individuals," *Vaccine* 32, no. 40 (2014): 5149–5155, doi: 10.1016/j.vaccine.2014.07.052.

271 "No Enigma: Vaccines and the Food Allergy Epidemic," Children's Health Defense, May 7, 2019, childrenshealthdefense.org/news /no-enigma-vaccines-and-the -food-allergy-epidemic.

272 Russell L. Blaylock, "A Possible Central Mechanism in Autism Spectrum Disorders, Part 1," *Alternative Therapies in Health and Medicine* 14, no. 6 (2008): 46–53, PMID: 19043938.

273 Alice E.W. Hoyt et al., "Alum-Containing Vaccines Increase Total and Food Allergen-Specific IgE, and Cow's Milk Oral Desensitization Increases Bosd4 IgG4 While Peanut Avoidance Increases Arah2 IgE: The Complexity of Today's Child with Food Allergy," *Journal of Allergy and Clinical Immunology* 137, no. 2 (2016): AB151, doi: 10.1016/j.jaci.2015.12.622.

274 Heather Fraser, *The Peanut Allergy Epidemic: What's Causing It and How to Stop It*, Third Edition, Skyhorse Publishing; 2017.

275 Margie Profet, "The Function of Allergy: Immunological Defense Against Toxins," *Quarterly Review of Biology* 66, no. 1 (1991), doi: 10.1086/417049.

276 "Vaxxed-Unvaxxed: The Science," Children's Health Defense, accessed Feb. 16, 2023, childrenshealthdefense.org/wp-content/uploads/Vaxxed-Unvaxxed-Parts-I-XII.pdf.

277 Stanislaw J. Gabryszewski et al., "Early-Life Environmental Exposures Associate with Individual and Cumulative Allergic Morbidity," *Pediatric Allergy and Immunology* 32, no. 5 (2021): 1089–1093, doi: 10.1111/pai.13486.

278 Chian-Feng Huang, Wei-Chu Chie, and I-Jen Wang, "Effect of Environmental Exposures on Allergen Sensitization and the Development of Childhood Allergic Diseases: A Large-Scale Population-Based Study," *World Allergy Organization Journal* 14, no. 1 (2021): 100495, doi: 10.1016/j.waojou.2020.100495.

279 "Food Allergies," Organic Consumers Association, accessed Feb. 21, 2023, organicconsumers.org/?s=food+allergies.

280 "The Truth Behind Allergies + Our Food Supply with Zen Honeycutt," Children's Health Defense, Dec. 13, 2021, live.childrenshealthdefense.org/chd-tv/shows/tea-time/the-truth-behind-allergies--our-food-supply-with-zen-honeycutt/.

281 Bénédicte Leynaert et al., "Does Living on a Farm during Childhood Protect against Asthma, Allergic Rhinitis, and Atopy in Adulthood?", *American Journal of Respiratory and Critical Care Medicine* 164, no. 10 Pt 1 (2001): 1829–1834, doi: 10.1164/ajrccm.164.10.2103137.

282 Sabina Illi et al., "Protection from Childhood Asthma and Allergy in Alpine Farm Environments—the GABRIEL Advanced Studies," *Journal of Allergy and Clinical Immunology* 129, no. 6 (2012): 1470-7.e6, doi: 10.1016/j.jaci.2012.03.013.

283 Josef Riedler et al., "Exposure to Farming in Early Life and Development of Asthma and Allergy: A Cross-Sectional Survey," *The Lancet* 358, no. 9288 (2001): 1129–1133, doi: 10.1016/S0140-6736(01)06252-3.

284 David Stukus, "Why It's Time to Rethink Our Use of Benadryl," Nationwide Children's, Apr. 9, 2020, nationwidechildrens.org/family-resources-education/700childrens/2020/04/benadryl.

285 "Epinephrine FDA Alerts," *Drugs.com*, Jan. 9, 2023, drugs.com/fda-alerts/989-0.html.

286 Bruce P. Lanphear, "The Impact of Toxins on the Developing Brain," *Annual Review of Public Health* 36 (2015): 211–230, doi: 10.1146/annurev-publhealth-031912-114413.

287 Benjamin Zablotsky et al., "Prevalence and Trends of Developmental Disabilities among Children in the United States: 2009–2017," *Pediatrics* 144, no. 4 (2019): e20190811, doi: 10.1542/peds.2019-0811.

288 Natalie A.E. Young, "Childhood Disability in the United States: 2019," United States Census Bureau, Report Number ACSBR-006, Mar. 25, 2021, census.gov/library/publications/2021/acs/acsbr-006.html.

289 "Data & Statistics on Autism Spectrum Disorder," Centers for Disease Control and Prevention, accessed Jan. 9, 2023, cdc.gov/ncbddd/autism/data.html.

290 Christine F. Delgado et al., "Lead Exposure and Developmental Disabilities in Preschool-Aged Children," *Journal of Public Health Management and Practice* 24, no. 2 (2018): e10–e17, doi: 10.1097/PHH.0000000000000556.

291 "NTP Study: 'Fluoride Is Presumed to Be a Cognitive Neurodevelopmental Hazard to Humans,'" Fluoride Action Network, Oct. 26, 2019, fluoridealert.org/content/bulletin_10-26-19.

292 *The Sickest Generation: The Facts Behind the Children's Health Crisis and Why It Needs to End*, second edition, Children's Health Defense, October 2020, childrenshealthdefense.org/ebook-sign-up/ebook-sign-up-the-sickest-generation.

293 Merideth Gattis, Alice Winstanley, and Florence Bristow, "Parenting Beliefs about Attunement and Structure Are Related to Observed Parenting Behaviours," *Cogent Psychology* 9, no. 1 (2022): 2082675, doi: 10.1080/23311908.2022.2082675.

294 "Attunement: The Beginnings of Human Play," National Institute for Play, accessed Feb. 27, 2023, nifplay.org/what-is-play/types-of-play/attunement-play.

295 Dawn Lee Garzon et al., *Burns' Pediatric Primary Care*, 7th Edition, Elsevier, 2019, bit.ly/3OfXaF9.

296 Kittie Butcher et al., "Why Crawl?", Michigan State University/MSU Extension, Mar. 15, 2013, canr.msu.edu/news/why_crawl.

297 "Learn the Signs. Act Early." Centers for Disease Control and Prevention, accessed Jan. 5, 2023, cdc.gov/ncbddd/actearly/index.html.

298 Jackie Spinner, "Developmental Milestones Just Changed for the First Time in Years," *Washington Post*, Feb. 10, 2022, washingtonpost.com/parenting/2022/02/10/new-developmental-milestones.

299 Jennifer M. Zubler et al., "Evidence-Informed Milestones for Developmental Surveillance Tools," *Pediatrics* 149, no. 3 (2022): e2021052138, doi: 10.1542/peds.2021-052138.

300 Steve Schering, "CDC, AAP Update Developmental Milestones for Surveillance Program," AAP News, Feb. 8, 2022, publications.aap.org/aapnews/news/19554/CDC-AAP-update-developmental-milestones-for.

301 Manuel E. Jimenez et al., "Access to Developmental Pediatrics Evaluations for At-Risk Children," *Journal of Developmental & Behavioral Pediatrics* 38, no. 3 (2017): 228–232, doi: 10.1097/dbp.0000000000000427.

302 Zablotsky et al., 2019.

303 Alia Wong, "Pandemic Babies Are Behind After Years of Stress, Isolation Affected Brain Development," *USA Today*, Jun. 9, 2022, updated Jun. 15, 2022, usatoday.com/in-depth/news/education/2022/06/09/pandemic-babies-now-toddlers-delayed-development-heres-why/9660318002.

304 "Early Identification of Speech, Language, and Hearing Disorders," American Speech-Language-Hearing Association, accessed Jan. 5, 2023,

asha.org/public/Early
-Identification-of-Speech
-Language-and-Hearing-Disorders.

305 "Find Certified Audiologists and
Speech-Language Pathologists
(SLPs)," American Speech-Language
-Hearing Association, accessed Aug. 1,
2023, asha.org/profind.

306 Georgia Chronaki et al., "The
Development of Emotion
Recognition from Facial Expressions
and Non-Linguistic Vocalizations
During Childhood," *British Journal of
Developmental Psychology* 33, no. 2
(2014): 218–236, doi: 10.1111/bjdp
.12075.

307 Svetlana Masgutova and Denis
Masgutov, "MNRI® Assessment
for Determining the Level of
Reflex Development," Svetlana
Masgutova Educational Institute for
Neuro-Sensory-Motor and Reflex
Integration, SMEI (USA), 2015,
masgutovamethod.com/the-method.

308 "What Are Cognitive Developmental
Delays," the Warren Center, accessed
Jan. 5, 2023, thewarrencenter.org
/help-information/cognitive/what
-are-cognitive-developmental
-delays.

309 Carolyn M. Gallagher and
Melody S. Goodman, "Hepatitis
B Vaccination of Male Neonates
and Autism Diagnosis, NHIS
1997–2002," *Journal of Toxicology
and Environmental Health*, Part A
73, no. 24 (2010): 1665–1677, doi:
10.1080/15287394.2010.519317.

310 Lanphear, 2015.

311 S. Feldman, "Immunization
Update," *Allergy Proceedings*
13, no. 6 (1992): 293–297, doi:
10.2500/108854192778816906.

312 Katie Weisman, "Just How Many
Shots Are on the CDC Schedule?",
Children's Health Defense, Dec. 7,
2017, childrenshealthdefense.org
/news/just-many-shots-cdc
-schedule.

313 F.T. Cutts, W.A. Orenstein, and R.H.
Bernier, "Causes of Low Preschool
Immunization Coverage in the
United States," *Annual Review of
Public Health* 13 (1992): 385–398, doi:
10.1146/annurev.pu.13.050192.00
2125.

314 Holly A. Hill et al., "Vaccination
Coverage among Children Aged
19-35 Months – United States,
2017," *Morbidity and Mortality Weekly
Report* 67, no. 40 (2018): 1123–1128,
doi: 10.15585/mmwr.mm6740a4.

315 Enrico Trigoso, "Toxic, Metallic
Compounds Found in All COVID
Vaccine Samples Analyzed
by German Scientists," *The
Defender*, Aug. 25, 2022,
childrenshealthdefense.org/defender
/toxic-metallic-compounds-covid
-vaccines-german-scientists.

316 Christopher Exley, "An Aluminum
Adjuvant in a Vaccine Is an Acute
Exposure to Aluminum," *Journal of
Trace Elements in Medicine and Biology*
57 (2020): 57–59, doi: 10.1016/j.jtemb
.2019.09.010.

317 José G. Dórea, "Integrating
Experimental (In Vitro and In Vivo)
Neurotoxicity Studies of Low-Dose
Thimerosal Relevant to Vaccines,"
Neurochemical Research 36, no. 6
(2011): 927–938, doi: 10.1007/s11064
-011-0427-0.

318 Kendra D. Stallings, Rebecca L.
Kitchener, and Nathaniel G. Hentz,
"A High-Temperature, High-
Throughput Method for Monitoring
Residual Formaldehyde in Vaccine
Formulations," *Journal of Laboratory
Automation* 19, no. 3 (2014): 275–
284, doi: 10.1177/2211068213504096.

319 Sin Hang Lee, "Melting Profiles May
Affect Detection of Residual HPV L1
Gene DNA Fragments in Gardasil®,"
Current Medicinal Chemistry 21, no. 7
(2014): 932–940, doi: 10.2174/09298
67321999140102110933.

320 D. Goldblatt, "Conjugate Vaccines,"
Clinical & Experimental Immunology
119, no. 1 (2000): 1–3, doi: 10.1046
/j.1365-2249.2000.01109.x.

321 Anthony Samsel and Stephanie
Seneff, "Glyphosate Pathways
to Modern Diseases VI: Prions,
Amyloidoses and Autoimmune
Neurological Diseases," *Journal of
Biological Physics and Chemistry* 17
(2017): 8–32, doi: 10.4024/25SA16A
.jbpc.17.01.

322 Noushin Heidary and David E.
Cohen, "Hypersensitivity Reactions
to Vaccine Components," *Dermatitis*
16, no. 3 (2005): 115–120, PMID:
16242081, pubmed.ncbi.nlm.nih.gov
/16242081.

323 Johannes J. Stelzner et al., "Squalene
Containing Solid Lipid Nanoparticles,
a Promising Adjuvant System for
Yeast Vaccines," *Vaccine* 36, no. 17
(2018): 2314–2320, doi: 10.1016/j
.vaccine.2018.03.019.

324 Gatti and Montanari, 2017.

325 "Components of mRNA Technology
'Could Lead to Significant Adverse
Events in One or More of Our Clinical
Trials,' Says Moderna," Children's
Health Defense, Aug. 6, 2020,
childrenshealthdefense.org/news
/components-of-mrna-technology
-could-lead-to-significant-adverse
-events-in-one-or-more
-of-our-clinical-trials-says
-moderna.

326 Peter N. Alexandrov, Aileen I. Pogue,
and Walter J. Lukiw, "Synergism
in Aluminum and Mercury
Neurotoxicity," *Integrative Food,
Nutrition and Metabolism* 5, no. 3
(2018), doi: 10.15761/IFNM.1000214.

327 G.S. Goldman, "Comparison of
VAERS Fetal-Loss Reports During
Three Consecutive Influenza
Seasons: Was There a Synergistic
Fetal Toxicity Associated with the
Two-Vaccine 2009/2010 Season?",
Human & Experimental Toxicology 32,
no. 5 (2013): 464–475, doi: 10.1177
/0960327112455067.

328 Sasha Latypova, "Intent to Harm –
Evidence of Conspiracy to Commit
Mass Murder by the US DoD, HHS
and Pharma Criminal Enterprise,"
Gold Standard Covid Science in
Practice – An Interdisciplinary
Symposium V: In the Midst of
Darkness Light Prevails, Session III:
Getting Away from the Control Grid,
Doctors for COVID Ethics, Dec. 10,
2022, doctors4covidethics.org
/session-iii-getting-away-from
-the-control-grid-2.

329 Ami R. Zota et al., "Reducing
Chemical Exposures at Home:
Opportunities for Action," *Journal of
Epidemiology and Community Health*
79, no. 9 (2017): 937–940, doi:
10.1136/jech-2016-208676.

330 "Phthalates Factsheet," Centers
for Disease Control and Prevention,
National Biomonitoring Program,
accessed Jan. 10, 2023, cdc.gov
/biomonitoring/Phthalates_Fact
Sheet.html.

331 "Flame Retardants
(Organophosphates) – OPs," Centers
for Disease Control and Prevention,
Division of Laboratory Sciences,
accessed Jan. 10, 2023, cdc.gov/nceh
/dls/oatb_capacity_03.html.

332 "Bisphenol A (BPA) Factsheet,"
Centers for Disease Control and
Prevention, National Biomonitoring
Program, accessed Jan. 10, 2023, cdc
.gov/biomonitoring/BisphenolA_Fact
Sheet.html.

333 "PFAS Explained," United States
Environmental Protection Agency,
accessed Jan. 10, 2023, epa.gov/pfas
/pfas-explained.

334 Sydney Evans and Katura Persellin,
"New Baby Textile Product Tests
Show Concerning Levels of Toxic
'Forever Chemicals,'" Environmental
Working Group, Nov. 3, 2022, ewg
.org/news-insights/news/2022/11
/new-baby-textile-product-tests
-show-concerning-levels-toxic
-forever.

335 Paul B. Tchounwou et al., "Heavy Metals Toxicity and the Environment," *Experientia Supplementum* 101 (2012): 133–164, doi: 10.1007/978-3-7643-8340-4_6.

336 "Health Effects of Lead Exposure," Centers for Disease Control and Prevention, Childhood Lead Poisoning Prevention, accessed Jan. 10, 2023, cdc.gov/nceh/lead/prevention/health-effects.htm.

337 "Chapter 1. Scope and Boundaries," United States Environmental Protection Agency, accessed Aug. 1, 2023, epa.gov/sites/default/files/2015-04/documents/wire_ch1.pdf, p. 3.

338 Tom Neltner, "Latest Federal Data on Lead in Food Suggests Progress Made in 2016 Was Fleeting," Environmental Defense Fund, Oct. 3, 2019, blogs.edf.org/health/2019/10/03/latest-federal-data-lead-food-progress-fleeting.

339 Greiner Environmental, Inc., *Environmental, Health and Safety Issues in the Coated Wire and Cable Industry*, University of Massachusetts Lowell, Technical Report No. 51, April 2002, turi.org/content/download/913/4501/file/Wire_Cable_TechReport.pdf.

340 "Chapter 1. Scope and Boundaries," United States Environmental Protection Agency, accessed Aug. 1, 2023, epa.gov/sites/default/files/2015-04/documents/wire_ch1.pdf, p. 3.

341 Kendra Pierre-Louis, "There's Lead in Your Christmas Tree Lights, But Is It Enough to Be a Serious Holiday Health Concern?", *Medical Daily*, Dec. 24, 2013, medicaldaily.com/theres-lead-your-christmas-tree-lights-it-enough-be-serious-holiday-health-concern-265735.

342 "Arsenic Factsheet," Centers for Disease Control and Prevention, National Biomonitoring Program, accessed Jan. 10, 2023, cdc.gov/biomonitoring/Arsenic_FactSheet.html.

343 Vladimir Bencko and Florence Yan Li Foong, "The History of Arsenical Pesticides and Health Risks Related to the Use of Agent Blue," *Annals of Agricultural and Environmental Medicine* 24, no. 2 (2017): 312–316, doi: 10.26444/aaem/74715.

344 "Mercury Factsheet," Centers for Disease Control and Prevention, National Biomonitoring Program, accessed Jan. 10, 2023, cdc.gov/biomonitoring/Mercury_FactSheet.html.

345 "Thimerosal in Vaccines Questions and Answers," U.S. Food & Drug Administration, Feb. 2, 2018, fda.gov/vaccines-blood-biologics/vaccines/thimerosal-vaccines-questions-and-answers.

346 "Thimerosal and Vaccines," U.S. Food & Drug Administration, Feb. 1, 2018, fda.gov/vaccines-blood-biologics/safety-availability-biologics/thimerosal-and-vaccines.

347 "Thimerosal in Vaccines Questions and Answers," FDA, 2018, bit.ly/3Km1bH4.

348 Cláudia S. Oliveira and Pablo A. Nogara, "Neurodevelopmental Effects of Mercury," *Advances in Neurotoxicology* 2 (2018): 27–86, doi: 10.1016/bs.ant.2018.03.005.

349 Oliveira and Nogara, 2018.

350 "Cleaning Up a Broken CFL: Recommendations for When a CFL or Other Mercury-Containing Bulb Breaks," U.S. Environmental Protection Agency, updated Jun. 9, 2023, epa.gov/mercury/cleaning-broken-cfl.

351 Christopher Exley, "Human Exposure to Aluminum," *Environmental Science. Processes & Impacts* 15, no. 10 (2013): 1807–1816, doi: 10.1039/c3em00374d.

352 Christopher Exley, "What Is the Risk of Aluminum as a Neurotoxin?", *Expert Review of Neurotherapeutics* 14, no. 6 (2014): 589–591, doi: 10.1586/14737175.2014.915745.

353 C.R. Casella and T.C. Mitchell, "Putting Endotoxin to Work for Us: Monophosphoryl Lipid A as a Safe and Effective Vaccine Adjuvant," *Cellular and Molecular Life Sciences* 65, no. 20 (2008): 3231–3240, link.springer.com/content/pdf/10.1007/s00018-008-8228-6.pdf.

354 Jason M. Glanz et al., "Cumulative and Episodic Vaccine Aluminum Exposure in a Population-based Cohort of Young Children," *Vaccine* 33, no. 48 (2015): 6736–6744, doi: 10.1016/j.vaccine.2015.10.076.

355 Exley, "An Aluminum Adjuvant in a Vaccine Is An Acute Exposure to Aluminum," 2020.

356 "Countries that Fluoridate Their Water," Fluoride Action Network, Apr. 7, 2021, fluoridealert.org/content/bfs-2012.

357 Tracy Connor, "Study Links Fluoridated Water During Pregnancy to Lower IQs," *Daily Beast*, Aug. 19, 2019, thedailybeast.com/fluoridated-water-during-pregnancy-linked-to-lower-iqs-study-published-by-jama-pediatrics-says.

358 Rivka Green et al., "Association Between Maternal Fluoride Exposure During Pregnancy and IQ Scores in Offspring in Canada," *JAMA Pediatrics* 173, no. 10 (2019): 940–948, doi: 10.1001/jamapediatrics.2019.1729.

359 John D. MacArthur, *Pregnancy and Fluoride Do Not Mix*, CreateSpace Independent Publishing Platform; 2016, pregnancyandfluoridedonotmix.com/thebook.html.

360 Morteza Bashash et al., "Prenatal Fluoride Exposure and Attention Deficit Hyperactivity Disorder (ADHD) Symptoms in Children at 6–12 Years of Age in Mexico City," *Environment International* 121, pt 1 (2018): 658–666, doi: 10.1016/j.envint.2018.09.017.

361 Atul P. Daiwile et al., "Role of Fluoride Induced Epigenetic Alterations in the Development of Skeletal Fluorosis," *Ecotoxicology and Environmental Safety* 169 (2019): 410–417, doi: 10.1016/j.ecoenv.2018.11.035.

362 Elise B. Bassin et al., "Age-Specific Fluoride Exposure in Drinking Water and Osteosarcoma (United States)," *Cancer Causes Control* 17, no. 4 (2006): 421–428, doi: 10.1007/s10552-005-0500-6.

363 "Fluoride Exposure and Human Health Risks: A Fact Sheet from the IAOMT," International Academy of Oral Medicine & Toxicology, updated Sep. 25, 2017, files.iaomt.org/wp-content/uploads/IAOMT-Fact-Sheet-on-Fluoride-and-Human-Health.pdf.

364 Christopher Exley, "Water Fluoridation: No Thanks, But Why?" *Dr's Newsletter*, Substack, Mar. 20, 2023, drchristopherexley.substack.com/p/water-fluoridation.

365 "Electric & Magnetic Fields," National Institute of Environmental Health Sciences, accessed Jan. 10, 2023, niehs.nih.gov/health/topics/agents/emf/index.cfm.

366 Michael Robb, "Kids' Screen Time Shifts Dramatically Toward Phones and Tablets," *Common Sense Media*, Oct. 18, 2017, commonsensemedia.org/kids-action/articles/kids-screen-time-shifts-dramatically-toward-phones-and-tablets.

367 "BioInitiative 2012: A Rationale for Biologically-based Exposure Standards for Low-Intensity Electromagnetic Radiation," Report Updated 2014–2022, bioinitiative.org.

368 "Cell Phones and Cancer Risk: Has Radiofrequency Radiation from Cell Phone Use Been Associated with Cancer Risk in Children?", National Cancer Institute, reviewed Mar. 10, 2022, cancer.gov/about-cancer

/causes-prevention/risk/radiation
/cell-phones-fact-sheet#has
-radiofrequency-radiation-from
-cell-phone-use-been-associated
-with-cancer-risk-in-children.

369 Merinda Teller, "Debunking
the Myth that Microwave Ovens
Are Harmless," Weston A.
Price Foundation, Nov. 5, 2019,
westonaprice.org/health-topics
/debunking-the-myth-that
-microwave-ovens-are-harmless.

370 *The Sickest Generation*, Children's
Health Defense, 2020, bit.ly
/3YotFpp.

371 Aviva Romm, "Who's Afraid of
Fever? An MDs Natural Approach to
Fever in Children," Avivaromm.com,
accessed Feb. 28, 2023, avivaromm
.com/natural-fever-treatments/#0
-fear-of-fever.

372 Sarah Pope, "Traditional Remedies
for Childhood Illnesses," Weston A.
Price Foundation, Mar. '22, 2009,
westonaprice.org/health-topics
/childrens-health/traditional
-remedies-for-childhood-illnesses.

373 *Anthromedics*, anthromedics.org.

374 "Acetaminophen—Not Worth the
Risk," Children's Health Defense,
Jul. 18, 2019, childrenshealthdefense
.org/news/acetaminophen-not
-worth-the-risk.

375 Michael Nevradakis, "Exclusive:
Hundreds of 'Tylenol Lawsuits'
Allege Retailers, Manufacturers
Knew Acetaminophen During
Pregnancy Could Cause Autism,
ADHD," *The Defender*, Jan. 11, 2023,
childrenshealthdefense.org/defender
/tylenol-lawsuits-acetaminophen
-pregnancy-autism-adhd.

376 Romm, "Who's Afraid of Fever?"

377 Erica Sweeney, "What Do Doctors
Mean When They Say 'Drink Plenty
of Fluids'?" Washington Post, Nov.
5, 2021, washingtonpost.com
/lifestyle/2021/11/05/what-do
-doctors-mean-when-they-say
-drink-plenty-fluids.

378 Elizabeth Pratt, "How Sleep
Strengthens Your Immune System,"
Healthline, Feb. 20, 2019, healthline
.com/health-news/how-sleep
-bolsters-your-immune-system.

379 Tom Cowan, "Fevers in Children,"
Weston A. Price Foundation, Nov. 12,
2005, westonaprice.org/health
-topics/ask-the-doctor/fevers-in
-children.

380 Philip Incao, "A New Attitude
Toward Fevers: An Interview with
Philip Incao, MD," *Pathways to
Family Wellness*, Issue 34 (Summer
2012), pathwaystofamilywellness
.org/Holistic-Healthcare/a-new
-attitude-toward-fevers-an
-interview-with-philip-incao-md
.html.

381 Natasha Campbell-McBride, *Gut
and Psychology Syndrome: Natural
Treatment for Autism, Dyspraxia,
ADD, Dyslexia, ADHD, Depression,
Schizophrenia*, 2nd Edition,
Medinform Publishing; 2010.

382 Romm, *Naturally Healthy Babies and
Children*, 2003.

383 *NAEYC*, naeyc.org.

384 Alice Callahan et al., "The Types of
Plastics Families Should Avoid," *New
York Times*, Apr. 18, 2020, nytimes.com
/article/plastics-to-avoid.html.

385 "Fact Sheet: Toys and Childhood
Lead Exposure," National Center
for Healthy Housing, Aug. 21, 2007,
nchh.org/resource/fact-sheet_toys
-and-childhood-lead-exposure.

386 Judy Frizlen, "Balancing Child Safety
and Risk in the Parenting Dance,"
LifeWays, 2016, lifewaysnorthamerica
.org/article_hidden/balancing
-child-safety-and-risk-in-the
-parenting-dance-by-judy-frizlen.

387 "Car Seats and Booster Seats,"
National Highway Traffic Safety
Administration (NHTSA), accessed
Jan. 14, 2023, nhtsa.gov/equipment
/car-seats-and-booster-seats.

388 "Learn First Aid for a Baby Who
Is Choking," British Red Cross,
accessed Jan. 10, 2023, redcross.org
.uk/first-aid/learn-first-aid-for
-babies-and-children/choking-baby.

389 Joel Streed, "Swallowed Objects and
Infant Choking: Tips for Parents and
Caregivers," Mayo Clinic, Jul. 31,
2013, newsnetwork.mayoclinic.org
/es/2013/07/31/swallowed-objects
-and-infant-choking-mayo-expert
-offers-tips-for-parents-and
-caregivers.

390 Simplicity Parenting,
simplicityparenting.com.

391 Debbie L. Stoewen, "Dimensions
of Wellness: Change Your Habits,
Change Your Life," *The Canadian
Veterinary Journal* 58, no. 8 (2017):
861–862, PMID: 28761196.

392 Michael R. Irwin, "Why Sleep
Is Important for Health: A
Psychoneuroimmunology
Perspective," *Annual Review of
Psychology* 66 (2015): 143–172, doi:
10.1146/annurev-psych-010213
-115205.

393 Theodore V. De Beritto, "Newborn
Sleep: Patterns, Interventions,
and Outcomes," *Pediatric Annals*
49, no. 2 (2020): e82–e87, doi:
10.3928/19382359-20200122-01.

394 Kelly R. Evenson et al., "Summary of
International Guidelines for Physical
Activity Following Pregnancy,"
Obstetrical & Gynecological Survey 69,
no. 7 (2014): 407–414, doi: 10.1097
/OGX.0000000000000077.

395 Jennifer Grafiada, "Nourishing
the New Mother: The Lost Art
of Postpartum Care," Weston A.
Price Foundation, Feb. 1, 2019,
westonaprice.org/health-topics
/womens-health/nourishing-the
-new-mother-the-lost-art-of
-postpartum-care.

NOTES

NOTES

NOTES

NOTES